SLEEP TRAINING

You Can Deal With It Effectively and Get
Happiness and Health Benefits

(Learn How to Adopt Healthy Habits and Adjust
Your Lifestyle)

Fannie Harvey

Published by Tomas Edwards

© **Fannie Harvey**

All Rights Reserved

Sleep Training: You Can Deal With It Effectively and Get Happiness and Health Benefits (Learn How to Adopt Healthy Habits and Adjust Your Lifestyle)

ISBN 978-1-990268-37-3

All rights reserved. No part of this guide may be reproduced in any form without permission in writing from the publisher except in the case of brief quotations embodied in critical articles or reviews.

Legal & Disclaimer

The information contained in this book is not designed to replace or take the place of any form of medicine or professional medical advice. The information in this book has been provided for educational and entertainment purposes only.

The information contained in this book has been compiled from sources deemed reliable, and it is accurate to the best of the Author's knowledge; however, the Author cannot guarantee its accuracy and validity and cannot be held liable for any errors or omissions. Changes are periodically made to this book. You must consult your doctor or get professional medical advice before using any of the suggested remedies, techniques, or information in this book.

Upon using the information contained in this book, you agree to hold harmless the Author from and against any damages, costs, and expenses, including any legal fees potentially resulting from the application of any of the information provided by this guide. This disclaimer applies to any damages or injury caused by the use and application, whether directly or indirectly, of any advice or information presented, whether for breach of contract, tort, negligence, personal injury, criminal intent, or under any other cause of action.

You agree to accept all risks of using the information presented inside this book. You need to consult a professional medical practitioner in order to ensure you are both able and healthy enough to participate in this program.

Table of Contents

Introduction

This book contains effective strategies on improving the way that you sleep immediately and with peace of mind. Discover proven, life-changing techniques to sleep better and finally get the sleep that you need!Sleep is absolutely essential for almost every single body function. In addition, it feels great as well! There are some common sleep disorders that many people face. Fortunately there are many simple things that we can do in order to enjoy a restful sleep.

Thanks again for downloading this book. I hope you enjoy it!

Chapter 1: Sleep Disorders From Apnea To Insomnia

Sleep itself is important for your mental and your physical wellbeing.Lack of sleep has many consequences that can make everyday life a struggle.Lack of restful, refreshing sleep is labeled as insomnia; however, many sleep disorders contribute to or even cause insomnia.

It is important to see a doctor if you have insomnia; sometimes correcting a pre-existing sleep disorder will relive the insomnia.

Anything that disturbs your sleep on a regular basis has the potential to cause insomnia.Snoring by you or your partner can cause insomnia; the constant disrupted sleep can eventually disrupt your sleep wake cycle and cause sever bouts of insomnia.

Correcting the snoring will remove the trigger that caused the insomnia, but you may still be left with insomnia itself.

Every sleep disturbance that occurs on a regular basis can trigger insomnia, if the disturbance continues for any period of time, and the insomnia continues, correcting the sleep disturbance may leave you to battle the insomnia it created.

Recognizing a sleep disturbance and correcting it quickly can eliminate the insomnia before it takes hold.

Understanding sleep disorders will help you eliminate triggers before they cause insomnia itself.

Sleep Apnea

Sleep Apnea is a huge problem that can go unnoticed for long periods of time.Two types of sleep apnea exist; central sleep apnea and obstructive sleep apnea.

Central sleep apnea is rare, bouts of central sleep apnea occur when the brain does not send the proper breathing signals and breathing becomes shallow or stops altogether.

Obstructive sleep apnea is the most common form of sleep apnea.Obstructive sleep apnea occurs because the airway restricts airflow because of a partial or complete collapse in the airway.The obstructed air way cuts off breathing and can cause snoring.

Both types of sleep apnea cause the patient to wake up several times during sleep.When the apnea occurs, the individual moves from deep sleep to light sleep because the brain sends wake signals to trigger the person to wake up and take a breath.

Sleep apnea can occur up to 100 times during an hour, the more it occurs the less restful sleep the individual will get.

Each time apnea occurs the body wakes up in an effort to restore the airflow.The constant disrupted sleep can eventually lead to insomnia.If you have apnea, or think you may have sleep apnea, seek a professional's help.

Apnea can be diagnosed through a sleep clinic and there are ways to live with apnea and sleep through the night.

Sleep Paralysis

Sleep paralysis occurs during the transition between sleep and wakefulness and the transition between wakefulness and sleep.During sleep, the brain signals a paralysis of the body to keep the body from moving during dreaming.

When sleep paralysis occurs, the individual becomes aware and awake but the body is still paralyzed.The body can remain paralyzed for seconds up to several minutes.

During sleep paralysis the individual may sense a presence near them, hallucinate, or experience a pressure on the body, as if someone or something is holding them down.

These fearful experiences occur because the mind is not really fully awake and it is still capable of creating a"dreaming"scenario.Individuals who experience these fearful episodes cannot react to them because the body is still paralyzed.This condition is not a serious one, but it is very disruptive to restful sleep.

Parasomnias

Parasomnia means abnormal sleep.There are several parasomnias identified by the medical field, and each one can disrupt sleep and cause a lack of restful, quality sleep.The following are the most common parasomnias diagnosed by sleep doctors.

Sleepwalking–Sleepwalking or somnambulism is a sleep disorder that causes individuals to get up and walk, and/or perform actions while sleeping.

This affects 4% of adults and is more common in children.Those who sleepwalk have no memory of what they did while sleepwalking.Sleepwalking occurs during deep sleep/non-REM and leave the individual with no recollection of the event

REM Sleep Behavior Disorder–This is more common in men aged 50 or over.During an episode of REM sleep behavior disorder, the individual will act out dreams, many dreams are violent in nature.

This disorder is dangerous for the individual who has it and their sleep partner.The usual paralysis that occurs before REM begins does not occur and the individual is able to act out the actions of the dream.

Nightmares–Dreams that are reoccurring, realistic, vivid, and frightening are considered nightmares.Most people experience nightmares sometimes, but nightmares become a parasomnia when it disrupts sleep on a regular basis.

Night Terrors–Night Terrors affect about 3% of adults, it is more common in children.Night terrors occur during non

REM sleep, the individual will wake up startled, frightened and disoriented/confused, and they have no memory of why.

Nocturnal Sleep Related Eating Disorder–This disorder involves an individual who sleepwalks and eats food.This can cause weight gain and is dangerous because the individual is not aware of what they are doing and are at risk of eating nonfood items, and items they are allergic to.

Bruxism –Bruxism is grinding the teeth.This condition is damaging to the teeth and the jaw.Those who have this condition can break, wear down, and even lose their teeth.

Sleep disorders keep sufferers from getting restful sleep, and they suffer from the effects of disruptive low quality sleep.Many of these conditions are medical and should be treated by qualified sleep doctors.If they are left untreated and undiagnosed their sleep suffers and the conditions can escalate.

All of these sleep disturbances can result in insomnia.Any long term sleep disturbance can lead to insomnia, once insomnia takes hold, it can linger even after the initial sleep disturbance subsides or is treated.

If you suffer from any of these sleep disturbances, it is important to seek treatment for any sleep disturbance.Once the sleep disturbance is diagnosed and treated, any lingering insomnia will respond to the 7 steps in this book.

Chapter 2: A Common Problem

You're not alone. The Centers for Disease Control and Prevention report that an estimated 50 to 70 million Americans suffer from lack of sleep. Worldwide, almost one quarter of the worlds working people experience difficulty sleeping.

Stress at work, family worries, financial woes and relationship problems are high on the list of reasons so many of us struggle to get the sleep we need. The CDC typifies difficulty sleeping as a public health problem, due to the impact of sleeplessness on society as a whole. Sleeplessness can be responsible for accidents (including those on the road and in the operating theatre) and serious occupational errors. Nodding off at inappropriate times (at work, at school, while driving) and trouble concentrating are common problems seen in those who aren't sleeping well at night.

It's also worrisome that a lack of sleep can lead to health problems in those suffering from it. Diabetes, obesity, hypertension and even cancer can be provoked by a lack of sleep.

Most people need between 7 and 9 hours of sleep each night, but since 1942, the amount of sleep most people in the United States get is only 6.8 (an hour less than the 1942 average). This point to a diminished quality of life for those who aren't getting adequate sleep.

But why? What is it that's keeping us up at night?

Stress

Researchers at the Harvard Business School and Sanford's Graduate School of Business recently published a report that found that workplace stress is responsible for as many as 120,000 deaths per year, in the USA alone. In addition, researchers identified a cost of up to $190 billion in health care expenses attending this dire statistic.

Our lives have not only become busier, but much more sedentary. This is particularly true of office jobs. Add to this the constant worry in our lives about everything from job stability to family integrity to bills waiting to be paid, and you have a recipe for health disaster.

However, stress is not always unhealthy. A little stress presses us forward, helping us get done what we need to get done and to achieve our goals. A completely stress-free life would bear little fruit. There's a line, though, and when that line is crossed, your sleep and health can be severely impacted.

When stress prevents us from resting adequately, there is a cascading effect in our lives. Irritability, depression, sluggishness and inattention can all lead to life consequences in our families, relationships and workplaces.

What's The Stress Point?

Your first move towards addressing stressors in your life that are preventing you from getting the rejuvenating rest you need, is to identify what's really eating away at you.

Researchers at KJT Group, Phillips, discovered that the most common stressors related to sleep problems were money and work. 28% of respondents in the study cited economic concerns as the factor that burdened them with the greatest amount of stress. 25% said work was their most stressful life reality.

This won't be news to many of us, but perhaps asking ourselves if these are the thoughts that keep us awake at night is a start. Sometimes, life's ups and downs are carried into our beds at night, preventing us from getting the rest we need.

Are you overtaxed at work? Do you have a physical pain issue? Is there a looming problem in your life you need to take positive steps toward addressing?

So What Should You Do About It?

• **Don't hold it in.** Talk to someone close to you. Taking the time to tell a friend or family member that something's bothering you can help to lighten your load. Take the time to write down the pros and cons of situations that may be bothering you. Be orderly in your financial affairs. Be diligent in living within your means, to the best of your ability. If your job is keeping you up at night, maybe it's not the right job for you. Taking stock of situations weighing on your mind is the first step toward addressing them effectively.

- **Make time for self-care.** Use your breaks at work to disengage from what you're doing. Go for a walk. Sit quietly somewhere and look out through the window. Go and get a cup of tea. If you can avoid it, don't work through your breaks. Take them and use them as your oases in a busy day.

- **Where does it hurt?** Go and ask your doctor if there's a health issue more serious than an ache or pain. Engage yourself in an activity that relieves the pain, like swimming or yoga (more on these below in the "Exercise" section).

Don't suffer in silence; it will only add to your stress. Share it with a professional who can help.

- **Be kind to yourself.** You are not a failure because you can't manage everything that gets piled on you. Maybe you're so accommodating that people come to you first when there's something they want done. Maybe it's time to address that. Learning to say "no", when appropriate to your needs and the work you're doing, is not a sign of weakness. It's an act of self-preservation. Embrace "no". Identify allies in your workplace willing and able to help and then, call on them.

- **Trouble on the home front?** Don't stew about it; act. Talk to your errant child, your irritable spouse, or whomever it is the problem is emanating from.Tell them how you feel.Not addressing the problem is causing it to grow in your mind, when it may be nothing at all, or something you can fix with a heart-to-heart, or the drawing of a boundary. Communication is your friend and leaves a better taste in your mouth than "stew".

• **Work smart, not hard:** One principle of effective time management is to do high quality work as opposed to high quantity work. The best way to do this is to concentrate on the results and not how busy you are. Just because you spend a lot of time, doing something does not mean that you will achieve better results. Similarly, staying an extra hour at your work may not be the best way to manage your time at the end of the day. Chances are you will feel resentful about working after hours. In addition, there is a high probability that you will be less productive, which will make you even more frustrated and compound your stress.

• **Do a good prep:** You'll have to admit that there's nothing stressful than being unprepared. You need to be organized for tomorrow, spend some time making your to do list and cleaning up before you leave. If you have everything covered up, you're less likely to fret about work when the night or evening comes. After you come in the following morning, you'll be relaxed to be in total control and able to handle things. Being prepared sets a positive tone for your day, and allows you to accomplish more things.

• **Prioritize:** Both men and women do worry but women tend to worry in a more global way. Men do worry on something specific or actual but women worry abstractly concerning their weight, job, or health status of a relative. However, try to keep your stress or worries focused only on real and immediate issues, and fight those that you have zero control on them.

Organizing your worries can help you reduce the stress overload.

• **Manage Your Time:** It's not unlikely and unheard of that you may get overwhelmed by the list of things you have to do. This may obviously be a cause of stress. It's a fact that you can't manage everything all at once unless you make schedules that are easy to follow. Begin by making a list of the things you want done based on priority. Also, categorize the list based on what you should do personally and what can be delegated to other people. Note those tasks that should be done immediately, those to be completed by the end of the day, next week or forthcoming week. The key here is to classify or manage big tasks into manageable tasks spread over some time, and delegating those that don't demand your personal attention. When managing your time, create buffer times where you can address emergency or unexpected tasks. Also have some time to relax and restore your well being.

● **Say 'No':** This is important when you have too much to do over a little period. Learn to say "No" to unimportant requests or additional tasks that can overwhelm you and cause stress. The sad thing is that majority of people can't manage to say "No" as they might appear rude and self-centered. However, be aware that barriers to this issue are self-created and can be overcome with a friendlier tone. Adopt a few humble expressions such as:

"I'd love to do this, but ..."

"I'm quite busy now. Can you ask me again at....?"

● **Take Control:** Some situations that cause worries, stress, and anxiety don't really mean that they are impossible to solve. Learn to look for remedies to your problems so as to feel in control and reduce stress. If unsure of how to begin, write down the problem and then brainstorm as many possible solutions as you can. Then pick each solution and analyze the good and bad side of it to realize the safest and reliable solution. Highlight each step that you require to undertake to solve the problem, i.e. what to do, how to do it, when to complete and who to be involved.

• **Keep a regular journal:** Synchronizing your body's sleep wake cycle is a very effective strategy to achieve good sleep. Set a fixed bedtime and wake up time to ensure you get the same amount of sleep every day, even on weekends. You can take a nap to make up for lost sleep, instead of waking up late in the morning. This way, you can cover up for lost sleep without interfering with the sleep-wake pattern. How do you know if you are getting enough sleep? If you find yourself awake before the alarm feeling focused and mentally sharp, then you have slept enough.

• **Have a lunch break**: Most busy people tend to work through lunch break in a bid to get more work done. This is generally not a good idea, and can even prove to be counterproductive. It is generally agreed that taking at least thirty minutes off from your work will improve your productivity in the afternoon. Taking a break gives you a chance to relax and take your mind off work. You can take this time to do some exercise or go for a walk. You will get back to your desk feeling rejuvenated with renewed focus and a new set of eyes. You can even plan your day using a midday break to help you break up your work into manageable bits.

● **Try the "4D" method**: Attempting to do all tasks requested through your email might at the end make you feel unproductive, frustrated, and tired. It has been shown that more and more workaholics today are experiencing some form of email stress. The first decision you make when you open an email is very crucial when it comes to addressing work addiction. To effectively manage this burden, you may want to use the "4 Ds" model to make your decision:

-Delete: You can probably delete almost half of the emails you receive immediately

-Do: This applies when the email is urgent or when it can be dealt with quickly

-Delegate: If someone else can deal with the email better

-Defer: Schedule some time to deal with the email if it requires longer action

All these problems are manageable with some reflection on your part. In the whirlwind of our busy lives, we too often pretend there's no time to reflect; for introspection. But this is one of those tales we tell ourselves to perhaps avoid those internal dialogues that need to be conducted.

How Much Sleep Do You Really Need?

Sleep is very important and everyone makes a conscious effort to get enough of it to feel fresh and less tired. However, you could be living a highly productive life or having an insanely busy schedule. With numerous responsibilities, you're forced to economize, slice up your working time and try to balance between tasks. Based on research, 90 percent of people can function better after 7-9 hours of sleep. A further 3 to 5 percent may function normally after less than 6 hours of sleep while only 1 percent of people sampled could manage less than 5 hours of sleep.

Most studies have shown that lack of sleep has a number of side effects. It disrupts normal body systematic functions right from metabolism to the immune system. Insufficient sleep can also trigger health conditions such as mood disorders, memory problems, attention deficit disorder, low fertility, obesity, and heart disease. On top of these physical symptoms, extreme fatigue can make you less alert and more prone to impulse behavior, memory lapses, and inability to fight stressors.

Apart from the medical problems, sleep deprivation makes you less efficient at work, and lowers your ability to solve problems, make decisions, communicate effectively, be innovative, and adapt to situations. Despite this, around 1 percent of the people can manage to work efficiently on about 4 hours sleep without serious side effects. "Short sleepers" are people who have genetic mutations that allow them to thrive in busy environments and work all through.

What matters is the amount of time you sleep within 24 hours as opposed to the sleep you average during the course of a night. If you cannot manage the 7-9 hours of sleep daily, you can choose to take a few 20-minutes naps while in the taxi, at work or other place. Even if the 7-9 hours of sleep are recommended for your physical health, remember to balance with the health of your career. In most times, you have a tough deadline to complete tasks and it's worth it to stay up late till it's done.

My rule of life?

Time is not something you have. It's something you make. It's worth your while to carve out at least an hour a day to tackle the little things we too often let slide. Instead of tuning out in front of the television, tune in to some of the life details crying out for your attention.

Busy.Busy. Busy.

Go here. Go there. Do this. Do that. Pick up the kids. Pick up the groceries. Pay the bills. Have a social life?

If you feel there aren't enough hours in a day, you're certainly not the only one.In our over-stimulated, 24/7 culture, it's increasingly difficult for people to slow down long enough to realize just how fast they're going.

Slowing down to take stock of things; to enjoy life, is something few of us make a point of finding time for.We are over-scheduled, overtaxed and worst of all, over tired.

But no matter how tired we are, so many of us have difficulty getting the quality sleep we need and our modern day "busyness" is a big part of the problem.

The hectic pace of our lives can come between our pillows and us. American sleep scientists have discovered that people who experience poor sleep quality often "sleep snack". When their bodies are given an opportunity to slow down, even for a moment, they doze off. Sleep-deprived, this clear message from their bodies is saying, "I need a good night's sleep!"

But brief periods of rest like "sleep snacks" don't solve the problem. They're no substitute for the good night's rest you need to be at your most alert and effective.

If You Can't Beat The "Busy", Manage It

Those of us who work at home are especially vulnerable to work invading other sectors of our lives. Where does work end and the rest of your life begin? For those who work at home, it's a tough call. Even those of us who leave our homes every day to go to work often don't park that part of our lives outside the front door when we walk through it at the end of the day. The emails keep coming. The phone keeps ringing. Loose ends demand tying up. In some ways, 21st Century communication portals have not made our lives easier. They've just made our work lives more able to intrude on time with family and friends.

Drawing boundaries is a balancing act. Telling those you work with you're not available after a certain hour is sometimes seen as a declaration of disinterest. Nobody wants to hear from their boss in the middle of the night, but sometimes it happens. Varied time zones, emergencies and contingencies happen at midnight just as often as they do at 4:30, or 5:00 pm, when you're ready to leave for the day. Beyond such urgencies, you are in charge. Drawing boundaries is a process that should begin as early in your working relationship as possible. Don't permit a situation that encroaches on your personal time to continue for months, or even years on end. Doing so is as good as telling your boss or co-workers it's OK with you.

It's not OK to expect you to be available 24 hours a day. Whenever possible, be clear about your boundaries in this respect.

Instead of accommodating every demand, try saying something like:

"Thanks for calling on me. I'll be on this first thing in the morning."

You've quietly drawn a line in the sand. At the same time, you've acknowledged the importance of the request with the kind of language you've employed. In addition, you've shown appreciation for the trust placed in you. Try it. It works.

The demands of others don't mean you're not in control of your time. You are. Slowing down is about more than drawing boundaries for others, though. You have to draw them for yourself, too. Take an honest look at how you spend the "spare" time you have. What do you do to relax?

Is it actually relaxing, or is it just one more thing keeping you plugged in, busy and frayed around the edges?

Does it keep you awake at night, as your mind struggles to shut down and sleep?

Time management is a discipline that can be applied to every area of your life. If done intentionally and with integrity, you'll find there's time in your day for everything you need to do, including spending time with your family and friends. There's even time for you.

Here are some life hacks to get you started:

If You Leave The House To Work:

• **Lay out your work clothes the night before**. Make sure everything you're taking from your closet is clean and ready to wear. This will prevent last minute scrambles to locate a tie with no stains on it, or a snag and run-free pair of pantyhose.

● **Coming home at night, change your clothes.** Put them in the closet if they're still good to wear. If not, put them in the laundry. How many Saturdays have you spent picking dirty clothes off the floor, because that's where you threw them when you came home? Get your partner and/or family in on the act. The time you spend picking up clothes and putting them where they're supposed to be is now yours.

● **Flaking out on the couch** is something most of us like to do sometimes, but laying there night after night, with the television watching over you as you look passively on is not only a waste of your time, it's another source of noise. So many of us turn the television on the minute we walk in the front door each evening. Advertisements, the superficial news cycle, meaningless reality shows – these are not enriching your life. Reduce your viewing time gradually. Choose what you'll watch. If there's nothing on you find appealing, turn the television off. Use the time you'd usually spend passively receiving information you don't need doing something you enjoy. Go for a walk! Visit with a friend! Take up a hobby! Using the time consumed by television to make space for the activities and people you love, will bring you greater peace and better rest.

- **Reduce the time you spend on social media.** As we all know, platforms like Pinterest and Facebook can consume countless hours of the time we need to slow down and get back in touch with what we love about our lives. Have a purpose when you open your social media account. Say what you want to say. Share what you want to share, but don't spend countless hours scrolling when you might be soaking in your tub, taking a much-needed, restorative bath. Start by scheduling and limiting your time. As you begin to wean yourself off these time-consuming activities, you'll find you've replaced them with options that serve you and your wellbeing much more effectively. Like television, there are many empty calories involved. Use the time you've been spending on social media for something that nourishes you, instead!

If You Work At Home:

Telecommuting is an option a growing number of people turn to. Conventional wisdom may lead us to believe that working from home frees more of our time. It's often the case, though, that working in the home is rife with distractions and opportunities to squander time. On the other hand, some who work from home log more hours and find it difficult to detach from their working lives.

Many of the life hacks mentioned above apply to people working at home just as readily, but here are a few specially tailored to those who telecommute:

- **Schedule yourself.** Get up at the same time each day and follow an agenda. You can always re-organize for contingencies, but sticking to an overall "shape" is a good way for stay-at-home workers to remain focused.

- **Make a list** of what you want to accomplish during the course of your day. You might want to do this the night before. That way, your goals are already set and you can hit the ground running.

- **Head off temptation** by being disciplined as to when and for how long you take your breaks. Take these often. The time you'd spend commuting, waiting for the bus, dressing for the office, packing a lunch – all this is time you can use to get away from your laptop and do something to clear your head (how about a little exercise?).

- **Don't procrastinate.** Meet your deadlines and complete your deliverables by resisting the urge to involve yourself in household matters in the time you've allotted for work. There is time for those, but not when you're working. Work when you've scheduled yourself to work. Attend to other matters when you've completed your work for the day.

Honestly assess how effectively and efficiently you manage your time and ask yourself what else you can tweak to clear away time to address details you normally can't seem to get to. There is time in your life. There is ample opportunity for you to "unbusy" yourself.

You just need to sit down, map out a course of action that fits your lifestyle and make the time. When you discover all those hidden hours, you'll be astounded. You'll also feel less taxed, stressed and pushed up against the wall, because you have become the master of your time. You've created the space you need to feel more relaxed about the demands of life.

You have taken back your time! Achieving this is crucial to feeling more centered in your life.

Chapter 3: Classification

DSM-5 criteria for insomnia

The DSM-5 criteria for sleep deprivation incorporate the following:

Overwhelming depression with slumber quality, connected with one (or more) of the accompanying side effects:

Trouble in onset of sleep. (In kids, this may show as trouble starting slumber without interventions of caregivers.)

Trouble keeping up slumber, described by regular arousals or issues coming back to rest after enlightenments. (In kids, this may show as trouble coming back to rest without parental figure mediation.)

Early-morning arousing with failure to return to rest.

Moreover, the slumber unsettling influence causes clinically noteworthy trouble or hindrance in social, word related, instructive, scholastic, behavioral, or other essential regions of working.

The slumber trouble happens no less than 3 evenings every week.

The slumber trouble is available for no less than 3 months.

The slumber trouble happens regardless of satisfactory time for slumber.

The sleep deprivation is worse clarified by and does not happen solely amid the course of an alternate slumber issue (e.g., narcolepsy, a breathing related slumber issue, a circadian mood slumber wake issue, a parasomnia).

The sleeping disorder is not attributable to the physiological impacts of a substance (e.g., a medication of misuse, a solution).

Existing together mental issue and restorative conditions don't enough clarify the transcendent dissention of a sleeping disorder.

COMORBIDITY AND CAUSES

Characteristically insomnia either co-exists with or is cause as a result of:

If any psychoactive drugs are used which include stimulants involving certain herbs, medications, nicotine, caffeine, amphetamines, cocaine, aripiprazole, methylphenidate, modafinil, MDMA or increased intake of alcohol.

If anti-anxiety drugs are withdrawn for example pain-relievers (opioids) or benzodiazepines.

Any heart disease

History of thoracic surgery

Disorders of respiratory system including disorders of nocturnal breathing and deviated nasal septum

Restless legs syndrome, which can result in slumber onset sleep deprivation (sleep onset insomnia) because of the discomforting sensations felt and the need to move the legs or other body parts to soothe these sensations

Periodic limb movement disorder (PLMD), which happens amid slumber and can result in arousals of which the sleeper is unconscious.

Pain/Torment, a harm or condition that causes agony can block a single person from discovering an agreeable position in which to nod off, and can also cause arousing.

Shifting of hormones, for example, those that go before periods and those amid menopause

Life occasions, for example, trepidation, stress, tension, mental or emotional pressure, work issues, money related anxiety, conception and mourning.

Gastrointestinal issues, for example, constipation or acid reflux.

Mental issue, for example, bipolar issue, generalized anxiety disorder, clinical depression, post traumatic anxiety issue, schizophrenia, dementia obsessive compulsive disorder, and ADHD

Unsettling influences of the circadian beat, for example, jet lag and movement work, can result in powerlessness to rest at a few times of the day and inordinate sluggishness at different times of the day. Chronic circadian rhythm disorders are portrayed by comparable symptoms.

Certain neurological issue, cerebrum injuries, or a past filled with traumatic mind injury.

Therapeutic conditions, for example, hyperthyroidism and rheumatoid arthritis.

Use of over-the counter or solution tranquilizers (soothing or depressant medications) can create bounce back insomnia.

Poor slumber cleanliness, e.g., clamor or over-utilization of caffeine.

An uncommon hereditary condition can result in a prion-based, lasting and, in the long run, lethal type of a sleeping disorder called fatal familial insomnia.

Physical activity. Activity induced sleep deprivation/ insomnia is basic in players as prolonged slumber onset latency.

Rest and sleep studies utilizing polysomnography have proposed that individuals who have interruption in their sleep have lifted night time levels of flowing cortisol and adrenocorticotropic hormone They likewise have a hoisted metabolic rate, which does not happen in individuals who don't have sleep deprivation yet whose slumber is deliberately disturbed amid a slumber study. Investigations of metabolism of brain via positron emission tomography (PET) outputs show that individuals with a sleeping disorder have higher metabolic rates by night and by day. The inquiry remains whether these progressions are the reasons or results of long haul insomnia.

Steroid hormones and insomnia

Studies have been led with steroid hormones and a sleeping disorder. Changes in levels of cortisol, progesterone in the female cycle, or estrogen amid menopause are corresponded with expanded events of sleep deprivation. Those with varying levels of cortisol regularly have insomnia for a longer term, where insomnia is due to onset of estrogen catalyzed by menopause, and progesterone is insomnia for a shorter term in monthly lapse of female cycle.

Cortisol

Cortisol is regularly considered the anxiety hormone in people, yet it is additionally the wakening hormone. Analyzing salivation samples, taken in the morning, has demonstrated that patients with insomnia wake up with essentially lower cortisol levels when contrasted with a control having normal resting patterns. Further studies have uncovered that those with lower levels of cortisol after arousing have poorer memory when compared to those with ordinary levels of cortisol. Studies help that bigger measures of cortisol discharged at night happens in case of primary insomnia. For this situation, medications identified with cooling state of mind issue or uneasiness, for example, antidepressants, would control the cortisol levels and help forestall insomnia.

Estrogen

Numerous postmenopausal ladies have reported changes in slumber routines since entering menopause that reflect insomnia side effects. This could happen due to the lower levels of estrogen. Lower estrogen levels can result in hot flashes, change in anxiety responses, or general change in the slumber cycle, which all could help sleep deprivation. Estrogen treatment and estrogen-progesterone mix supplements as a hormone substitution treatment can help direct menopausal ladies' slumber cycle again.

Progesterone

Low levels of progesterone all through the female period cycle, however significantly near the end of the luteal stage, have additionally been referred to be connected with insomnia and peevishness, aggression and irritability in women. Around 67% of ladies have issues with sleep deprivation just before or amid their menstrual cycle. Lower levels of progesterone can, in the same way as estrogen, associate with insomnia in menopausal women.

A typical misperception is that the measure of slumber decrease as an individual ages. The capacity to rest for long stretches, instead of the requirement for slumber, gives off an impression of being lost as individuals get more established. Some elderly sleep deprived or insomniac people toss and turn in bed for whole night, reducing the measure of slumber they receive.

Hazard factors

Individual of all ages are effected by insomnia however individuals in the groups mentioned below have a higher shot of gaining a sleeping disorder.

People more than 60 years of age

History of mental illness including depression, and so forth.

Emotional anxiety

Working late night shifts

Traveling through distinctive time zones

Chapter 4: Finding The Best Sleep

One of the simplest and most important factors in a good nights sleep are the simple tools we use to sleep on. It has long been discussed exactly what texture of pillow is appropriate for the most restful sleep at night. A study done in Germany suggested that a pillow should be of a medium firmness in order to provide the best night sleep. Even though the exact firmness of a comfortable pillow will most likely vary depending on the person, the logic is sound. A pillow that is too soft causes a person to be engulfed by the pillow and forcing a person to ingest any pathogenesis or unhealthy substances that might be a part of the pillow. Even though a extremely firm pillow has not had any added benefit it could provide more comfort for some.

It makes sense that a pillow can often be the cause of many allergies and impaired breathing during the night. As over time they collect dust mites and certain allergens. It is common to have a down allergy. One of the best cures for these problems is to buy a non allergenic foam pillow and use a dust-mite proof covering. Running any pillow in the dryer will also kill and get rid of dust-mites. This should be practiced every couple of months to help keep your sleeping quarters healthy so that a restful night of sleep can be found by you each and every day.

The mattress in that you sleep on is another problem in finding the best night's sleep. In researching this book there is truly a study that will back up almost any kind of mattress.One study will say that foam mattresses are good where another will say they cause back pain. There are a lot of different types mattresses on the market today. The best advice is to choose the one that you are most comfortable sleeping on.

A mattress should be replaced every 8 to ten years because any longer than that the materials inside the mattress might start to degrade and cause poor sleeping posture and result in personal pain. This will deprive a person of sleep.The same time frame should be monitored for a box spring as well because over time it will lose a lot of its bounce and needs to be replaced.

When buying a mattress, comfort should be the major goal, because a comfortable sleeping environment will allow you to sleep better. Learning to shop for a mattress is a skill. Spend some extra time in the store and at least test the potential mattress for 15 minutes at least resting on the side of the bed that you would sleep on and in your preferred sleeping position.That way the reaction of your body to the mattress will not be a mystery to you.If the store allows for a sleep test, then take it seriously.

Talk to a chiropractor about the type of mattress that might conform to your body the best. Many believe that it is good to have a mattress that moves with the natural viticulture of your spine. This will make sure that your sleep is interrupted less and a better night's sleep can be achieved.

Chapter 5: Alternative Treatments And Home Remedies For Sleep Apnea

For most patients who suffer from sleep apnea, changes in the lifestyle is the best cure, so you should first try some home remedies and pay extra attention to your overall lifestyle.

Among the changes you can make in order to cure or ease your sleep apnea, no matter what type, are losing weight, quitting smoking and leading an active life.

Obesity and being overweight can trigger obstructive sleep apnea, as the throat gets coated in fat layer and the space available for air to pass by, shrinks. A basic loss of five to ten pounds will make some room and can ease your apnea or cure it completely.

Giving up on bad habits like smoking and binge drinking can also help you with this sleep condition, as both of these substances irritate the tissues and promote general inflammation.

If you take sleeping pills, you must know they can be blamed for your apnea, as these drugs relax the muscles and make the tissues go down more than in usual sleeping state. However, before giving up on them, ask your doctor's advice, as some need to be quit over time, by adjusting the dosage.

If you are living the modern, laptop-focused sitter life, get out there and move your muscles. Exercise, even as little as a 30-minute session, work great on toning up your body and can ease the sleep apnea by increasing the blood flow and the oxygen level in your body. A brisk walk or working out sometimes on the treadmill are enough to ease your symptoms in mild cases. If you regularly exercise for a week, you can see the results

As allergies can cause inflammation of your throat, you can use saline water or antihistamines to reduce the inflammation and keep the airways open. If you go for the natural method and use aromatherapy, acupuncture or saline mixture, you can follow your routine in long term, but antihistamines only work for short periods, like the spring weeks. If you go for using essential oils, marjoram, neroli, lavender and valerian are good picks, as they help reduce the inflammation and relax the tissues, which can sometime be all that is needed for sleep apnea. When you try these for the first time, make sure you are not alone and assess their effectiveness before you go for another dose, as you might worsen your sleep apnea.

Chapter 6: How To Have Lucid Dreams: Effective Techniques

Yes, lucid dreaming feels almost magical for many of us. This leads them to think that it is a difficult thing to learn. In reality, there are no complicated processes involved in learning how to have lucid dreams. Everybody can learn it. Basically, it is a skill that can be developed and gained through practice. Some of us have this capacity to easily go into lucid dreams. Some of us will experience it only by chance. Can you easily remember what you have dreamed about? If your answer is yes, this is good news as it is a success indicator for those who are planning to train in lucid dreaming.

Even if you don't have that natural talent to go into lucid dreams, you can successfully train for it. Your success will depend upon two very important factors. These include your motivation for the training and the amount of effort that you will put into the whole thing. Through the process of experimentation, observation, and continuous perseverance on training, positive results can be fast tracked.

The following techniques are proven to help individuals like you to have lucid dreams with ease:

TECHNIQUE #1: Recall of Dream Details – There are detailed steps that could be accessed from book EWLD (Exploring the World of Lucid Dreaming). However, the basic idea behind this technique is that you should develop the habit of immediately recording the details of your dreams by note taking. This is done immediately after waking up.

TECHNIQUE #2: Verification of Reality - This is a set of exercise that involves testing elements in your environment to see if there are impossible events that are happening. As an example, you could use your cellphone as a tool to tell time. Look at it and note the time. Look away for a few seconds and see if there will be impossible changes that would happen on the numbers, time, or even text.

TECHNIQUE #3: Identification of "Dream Signs" - This technique has its roots in the EWLD and has been further given attention in other related books. This technique trains you to study your dreams and its detailed elements. Signs that you are dreaming could be easily identified. Examples include a flying house, talking cats, or a never-ending road. You can remind yourself before sleeping that if you see these in your dreams, you'll be reminded that you are in a state of lucidity.

TECHNIQUE #4: The MILD Method – MILD means Mnemonic Induction of Lucid Dreams. On this technique, you will train yourself to remember to do a specific set of action once you have achieved lucidity. You will do this after being awakened from a dream and right before you return to sleep. It consists of three steps:

Setting up a dream that you want to recall

Concentrating on your intent to recall everything in the dream you just had

Voluntary induction to lucidity by thought suggestion and use of dream signs

TECHNIQUE #5: Planned and Timed Napping – There are two approaches on this technique that you can do. First, aim to have lucid dreams during the afternoon.

Your chances of success will be higher than when taking morning naps. Another approach is to interject wakefulness periods within your normal periods of sleeping during the night. It works like this:

Wake up an hour earlier from your normal waking time.

Stay up for at least 30-60 minutes while doing technique 1, 2, 3, and 4.

Resume sleeping.

The success that you'll get from these techniques will vary depending on your dedication to attaining gradual results and on the consistency of your training. Now that you have learned techniques in achieving lucid dreams, it is time for you to move on to sleep meditations. The next chapter will give you all the pertinent sets of information about it.

Chapter 7: Strategies To Tackle Stress

If you trace back each sleep disorder deep enough, you'll discover that most of them are more or less related to the two constituents that govern our sleep, i.e. homeostasis and circadian rhythm. One of the biggest factor that has a profound influence over the brain's hormones is stress. If you can beat the stress, half your problems will be easily wiped off. Stress is one of the direct causes of insomnia and plays a huge role in worsening one's sleep deprivation.

So the first thing you do is go head to head against stress and slowly yet surely throw it out of your life. So here's how you can put off that giant weight off your shoulders:

Exercise:

Exercise seems to be the answer to everything, doesn't it? It is by no coincidence that exercise or any kind of physical activity provides a solid relief from stress. It has been found that no matter how professional a person is at his/her job, he/she cannot excel in it until he/she eliminates stress & tension from his life. Stress is not only responsible for problems in your subconscious but can also disrupt your day to day activities. Going into the details of any specific exercise plan won't benefit anyone as there are hundreds of regimens, each with their own pros & cons. However, here's a general direction as to what you should adopt.

- Walking, running or jogging is one of the most effective exercises in the world. You can make it a part of your daily life simply by waking up early either on weekdays or by reserving time for them on weekends. You should look for a park or a natural environment for carrying out this activity. It is recommended that indoor gyms and treadmills be avoided. A few interactions with nature will bring back serenity in your life in addition to giving your body a physical makeover. Just 30 minutes of walk on alternate days would be enough.

- Go out for a swim if you have access to a swimming pool or there's a pond nearby. Once again this will illicit physical activity which would result in the release of "feel good" hormones in the brain.

- If you get tired of doing the same thing over and over again, i.e. walking then shift your focus to some kind of sport. Walking was mentioned here as it doesn't require that much time but if you have time to spare at the weekend then its best to join a sports club and get on with more interesting things.

- Last but not the least, join a gym. I'm not overly enthusiastic about the idea of a gymnasium unless it's an open air one as closed environments are what cause stress to develop in the first place so a natural environment would be much more better. But nevertheless gyms are great places when it comes to enhancing your social circle and talking can resolve a lot of issues. Give it a try if everything else doesn't suit you.

But what is the significance of exercise in all this? I bet you don't the answer to this. Well, here it goes; when the body engages in a physical activity, it stimulates endorphins that are pumped right into the bloodstream. Endorphins are the "feel good" chemicals that can give your brain an overhaul and a pleasant feeling for some time. That's not the end of it. Endorphins play a much wider game. They can impact the health of the central nervous system as well as the immune system as well. So exercise is not limited to giving you an empty head at night, it does much more.

Take Control:

Stress is something that can't be totally eliminated through biological remedies unless & until you decide to get a hold of your life. How can you do that, here's how:

- **Say "no"**: Stop being a pushover and put yourself ahead of others. This may sound a little self-centered but the truth is most people you deal with are almost looking out for themselves, except family and friends. You must realize the facts that you can't keep everyone happy so the next time someone asks you to do something due to which you'll have to put down your own preference, simply say no.

- **Duck people who are a source of tension**: All of us know people in our lives who are a constant source of worries; sometimes they are our friends, colleagues or people who we have to deal with every day. The best case scenario would be to terminate your relation with such a person, as nothing can top off your health but if that's not possible, then its best to limit your contact and who knows, maybe soon enough he/she will understand.

- **Look around:** If it is everyday news that drives you crazy, then turn the T.V off; if it's the traffic that riles you up in the morning, then take a longer yet less congested route or even better, take a bus which would give you a chance to socialize. If, like some people you hate to shop from store-to-store then shop online. These are just a few examples of how you can counter anxiety by eliminating the little stressors in your life.

Alter the Situation:

Sometimes things go so fast that giving up seems the most viable choice. If you're feeling like that with the above strategies then shift to the one day at a time approach. Changing the current scenario is the easiest thing you can do to tackle stress:

- **Be expressive**: The may sound as a daunting task especially for men but the truth is that expressing your feelings can let out a lot of steam. This can cool you up from the inside and induce feelings of satisfaction within the mind & body. Communicate with your friends/partner in a more assertive, open yet respectful manner. Bottling up your feelings would only mount up pressure in your head until one day you ruin everything you've worked so hard for.

- **Compromise**: Just like you, the other person has ego and self-respect as well. Don't expect the person next to you to submit to your will. Give respect to get respect. Try your best to negotiate a settlement rather than scaling a full on offensive, whether it's a domestic issue or something at work.

- **Manage**: Build a simple and comprehensive timetable for all your daily tasks. Putting your life in order can take a lot of stress and haphazardness out of everyday activities. If you have a proper organized schedule then you would do each task with full dedication rather than impatiently moving on the next one. Most people miss out on deadlines due to the simple fact that they failed to plan ahead before starting off the project. So the best thing to do is to set up a simple schedule for your everyday activities; and remember you don't need to track every minute of your time, just an overall view would be enough.

Chapter 8: Breathing Devices For Sleep Apnea

The case of those with severe sleep apnea is different. Self help strategies may not suffice for successful treatment.

Before an appropriate treatment can be decided on, the patient needs to see a doctor and a sleep specialist. These professionals will work at evaluating the symptoms which can help them arrive at an effective treatment.

The treatment options for complex and central sleep apnea vary. But they typically include the treatment of any underlying medical condition first that may cause the sleep apnea. These conditions may include neuromuscular disorder or heart disease.

Complex and central sleep apnea are usually treated using supplemental oxygen during sleep or breathing devices. Such may also be used for the treatment of obstructive sleep apnea. Medications may be prescribed but only in cases of sleepiness in connection with apnea.

CPAP for Sleep Apneics

Known as the most common treatment for both moderate and severe cases of obstructive sleep apnea, CPAP or Continuous Positive Airflow Pressure involves the use of a mask-like machine providing a continuous stream of air. This helps apneics keep their breathing passages open during sleep. This device is typically as big as a box of tissue.

The air pressure provided by the CPAP device is somewhat greater than the surrounding air. It is not just the most common treatment for sleep apnea, it is also considered as the most reliable. By keeping the upper airway passages of the patient open, CPAP can prevent snoring and apnea episodes.

While many patients are satisfied with the CPAP device, it is also common for patients to find wearing it uncomfortable. This device definitely needs some getting used to. When the mask straps are properly adjusted to provide a more secure fit, you may find it less cumbersome to wear. In some cases, patients may be advised to use a humidifier and the CPAP system at the same time.

Tips for Adjusting to a CPAP Unit

It is completely natural to miss your old way of sleeping. It is natural to feel that the mask is more of an obstruction rather than help. But the truth is many people find it effective. And it is definitely worth the try. It may take some adjustment though. That said below are some tips to help you adjust easily to your CPAP mask.

First, check on proper fit. Many people who find the mask troublesome are wearing a mask that does not provide a secure fit. The mask should neither be too loose nor too tight. You can check on the straps to ensure you have it on just right.

Second, allow an ease in period. You do not have to force yourself to like wearing the mask. Again, it is okay to feel weird about having to wear a mask to sleep. Start by wearing it for only short periods throughout the day. You can also utilize the ramp setting which can help you increase the air pressure in a gradual manner. Normally, people require several months before they feel comfortable sleeping with the CPAP device on. So, you do not have to feel bad about it.

Third, customize the device. You can actually have the device customized. Components of the CPAP machine including the straps, mask and the tubing can be customized to provide you with the best fit possible. There are also available soft pads. These pads can help in reducing skin irritation as a result of wearing the device. You can also get nasal pillows and chinstraps which may help lessen the chances of throat irritation.

Fourth, try it with a humidifier. Some patients complain about skin irritation and dryness when using the CPAP machine. Another effective way to avoid such things is to use a humidifier along with the machine. A special moisturizer may also be applied before going to bed. In fact, latest models of CPAP are now equipped with a built-in humidifier.

Fifth, keep your CPAP machine clean. Another simple way of preventing skin dryness and irritation is to ensure the tubing, mask, and headgear are kept clean. Using a humidifier can also help ensure this.

Sixth, you can also quiet the CPAP unit down. If you find the sound coming from the machine bothersome, you have the option to position it under the bed. Using a sound machine may also help. The features of CPAP machines are constantly adjusted. Now there are CPAP machines that are made to be lighter and quieter.

Finally, if you really find the CPAP mask irritable, you can also give the alternative a try. This alternative is called Provent. It is CPAP without the mask. Instead, patients are provided with a device small enough to fit the nostrils. It could be a more comfortable option but it is also usually more expensive.

Other Breathing Devices Recommended for Sleep Apneics

Sleep specialists may also recommend other breathing devices. Such recommendations may include BPAP and ASV.

BPAP or Bilevel Positive Airway Pressure

This can be used as an alternative option to CPAP especially or patients who find it difficult to adjust to the CPAP unit. BPAP can prove helpful especially to individuals suffering from central sleep apnea who have a weak breathing pattern.

The BPAP is designed to adjust the air pressure automatically as the patient sleeps. When the patient inhales, the device provides more pressure. And when you the patient exhales, the device adjusts and provides less air pressure. There are BPAP devices that are designed to help the patient breathe again when the unit detects the patient has not taken a breath for several seconds.

ASV or Adaptive Servo-Ventilation

Targeted for individuals with central and obstructive sleep apnea, ASV devices can monitor and store information about the patient's normal breathing pattern. It is made to deliver airflow pressure which is meant to prevent breathing pauses which is one of the potentially dangerous symptoms of the condition.

Chapter 9: Time Management And Sleep

About Time Management

In the previous chapters, you were exposed to a heap of information about sleep. Now, you are familiar with its health benefits, as well as the health risks that are associated with sleep deprivation. By now, you understand that sleep is seamlessly linked to proper brain function, weight loss, muscle building, emotional health, and much more. In essence, your body could not function without sleep.

The next step in the process is to start putting sleep promotion skills into action. There are a few major causes behind sleep deprivation, and this book will assess each of them. The issues that generally impair one's ability to sleep include time management, lifestyle and environment, and nutrition and physiology.

One of the most commonly reported reasons for voluntary sleep deprivation are improper time management. Sometimes, sleep deprivation is rationalized amid a demanding career, the obligations of child rearing, relationships, projects, school, exercise, and socializing. With this said, many people sleep for under six hours per night in order to accommodate each of these critical responsibilities. However, as you learned, sacrificing a single night of sleep can raise blood pressure, increase stress and fat storage; promote muscle loss and much more.

If you want to reap all of the benefits of achieving a healthy sleep cycle, then it is crucial that you prioritize these time management techniques. As you will note, one of the most critical facets of engaging in healthy sleep patterns is time management. Without time management, you will not be able to balance your demanding life with healthy sleep habits. Failure to manage these techniques will lead to one of two results. You will either sleep too much at the expense of your family life, career and relationships, or you will deprive yourself of sleep in order to attend to your other responsibilities. Read below in order to learn more about time management skills.

Tip 1: Prioritize Important Tasks

Some people lament that there is never enough time during the day to attend to their most profoundly important responsibilities. However, one of the most common reasons behind this is that they do not prioritize their most important tasks first. If you want to balance sleep with socializing, relationships, family, career and school, you must prioritize important tasks first. In the beginning of the day, it is highly recommended that your important tasks take precedence over others. Once you have completed those tasks, you will be able to move onto more important ones, which you will have the option of postponing for the next day. When you take care of your most important tasks first, you will not fall prey to sacrificing sleep to attend to your important responsibilities. When you embark upon your most important tasks first, this leaves you time to prepare for sleep.

Tip 2: Say No When Necessary

Another critical means of maximizing your time is saying no when necessary. Taking on unnecessary commitments or socializing when you know it is unwise will hijack your time, and leave you susceptible to a sleepless night filled with procrastinated projects. The more you learn to master your life and take on commitments wisely, the more you will be able to improve the quality of your sleep and optimize your time.

Tip 3: Sleep

This seems rather counterintuitive, especially considering that this chapter is on time management techniques designed to increase your sleep. However, if you sleep between 7-8 hours at night, you will be more productive the following day. Hence, the more you sleep, the more you will accomplish during the following day. And the more you accomplish the next day in a timely fashion, the more you will be able to sleep that night as well.

Tip 4: Invest Yourself Fully In Your Current Task

Sometimes, people are so disgruntled with the task at hand that this detracts from their level of concentration and focus. When this occurs, they become less efficient and less productive, as well. The less efficient you are, the less time you will have to attend to your tasks. This makes the possibility of a sleepless night more likely. Give every project your all and you will maximize your time and sleep more later on.

Tip 5: Start Early

If you want a head start for sleep at night, then get a head start on your day. The earlier you get started, the more time you will have to balance work, school, sleep, family and social life.

Tip 6: Avoid unnecessary Details

Do not succumb to the bane of perfectionism! If you immerse yourself in irrelevant details, your tasks will take twice as long, leaving you less time to prioritize your health.

Tip 7: Make Your Responsibilities Your Habits

Many people see their most critical responsibilities, including work projects, as obligations. Try your best to turn these into habits, and make them a seamless part of your daily routine. Hence, when you complete the tasks, you will go about them naturally, with ease. The more habitual a task becomes, the more natural it feels. The more natural it feels, the less time it takes. This equates to more sleep for you.

Tip 8: Reduce Device Use

TV, gaming devices, smartphones and tablets all serve a critical function in today's age. Furthermore, they offer people endless hours of entertainment. In spite of this, excessive use of these devices can waste valuable time during the day. And when this occurs, it leaves one susceptible to procrastination and sleepless nights spent making up for lost time.

Tip 9: Set Deadlines

Time yourself during a task, and set a specific deadline. You can do this without compromising the quality of your work, as long as you invest yourself in what you are doing. If you delineate a set time frame for a task, you will work more productively, and you will be able to control the amount of time that you spend on your tasks. Once again, this equates to more sleep for you.

Tip 10: Take Breaks

The human body is a sensitive machine, and it is important to take breaks in between projects and obligations in order to rejuvenate our energy and motivate us for the next task. If you proceed from one task to the next, this will affect the quality of the work that you do and you will be less productive.

Tip 11: Think About One Task at a Time

If you obsess about every single task that you must perform on your to do list, you will feel very overwhelmed and spend more time worrying about your to do list than actually doing the work itself. When this happens, it makes you more susceptible to procrastination and sleepless nights. If you master one task at a time, you will complete all of your tasks with more mastery and efficiency.

Tip 12: Exercise

Exercise can offer you a much needed surge in energy, one that propels you forward throughout the day and gives you a much needed boost during tasks. Why is this? Because exercise leads to stimulation of your most vital functions which includes your cardiovascular system, this heightens your ability to function during the day.

Tip 13: Do Fewer Tasks

If you commit yourself to a few essential tasks each day, you can leave enough room for your relationship, family life, sleep, exercise, etc.

Tip 14: Productive Weekends

Weekends are not solely reserved for laziness and thoughtlessness. Even if you reserve 2-4 hours each weekend for productivity, you can lighten the load for the following week, and give yourself more time to engage in healthy sleep patterns. For instance, you can use these 2-4 hours on the weekend to pay bills, do grocery shopping, wash your car, handle errand, and clean, and reserve the rest of the week for important responsibilities such as your work life and personal life.

Tip 15: Remove Yourself from Distracting Environments

Distractions have a tendency to make people procrastinate and work through sleepless nights. When this happens, it is very important that you remove yourself from those distractions so that you will have time for your work and health.

Tip 16: Make Good Commitments

Commit to responsibilities that are meaningful to you and those that will take you to the next level. Do not take on unnecessary tasks.

Tip 17: Do Similar Things All At Once

Suppose you have to do laundry and mop during the day. These are fairly similar tasks that you can lump together in a single cleaning session. While your clothing is washing in the washer, you can mop and complete the tasks extra fast.

Tip 18: Reserve an Hour before Bed To Get a Head Start

This is fairly logical. The more time you have to relax before bed, the better your sleep will be.

Tip 19: Balance Tasks with Others

Is there someone in your life who can take a load of stress off of you? Contrary to popular belief, you do not have to do it all.

If you are engrossed in a critical work project, why not ask you significant other to handle dinner or a few errands if they are not busy? If you are burdened with school perhaps your roommate can do the chores this time? Try to allocate responsibilities in a fair and equitable fashion, and you will have more time to rest at night.

Tip 20: Prepare Meals in Advance

If you live alone, then you most likely prepare your own meals. If this is the case, then you most likely understanding how time consuming this is. One way to maximize your time during the day is to prepare your meals in advance.

Tip 21: Exercise before Work

By the time you work day is over, you are probably far too fatigued to exercise. When this happens, you are more likely to work out late, and compromise your ability to sleep in a healthy fashion. Wake up extra early. Not only will this help you fit in an extra workout, but it will help you go to bed at a more reasonable time. The earlier you wake up, the earlier you can go to bed.

Tip 22: Exercise during Work

Some professional settings are equipped with gym equipment. If your job doesn't have a gym, there are workouts that you can do right in the comfort of your office. This will save you time so that you can sleep at night.

The Super Schedule

Continue reading to learn more about the super schedule. This schedule is designed for those who truly want to be superhuman. What this means is that if you are serious about balancing all of the most important aspects of your life together, you truly can attend to the most valued aspects of your life by scheduling like a pro.

What is the secret to creating an amazing schedule, one that will help you accommodate all of your greatest needs? If you are an exceedingly busy person, then you have most likely experience sleep deprivation at some point. In life, it is difficult to balance your needs with your wants. Even though you need to exercise, work, complete projects and run errands, you want to spend time with your kids or significant other, go on dates, socialize, watch TV and relax.

The key to mastering time and developing a super scheduler is to balance what you need with what you want. You should never eliminate all of your wants from daily schedule. However, it is important to complete the urgent needs during that day, and reserve time for select wants. The following list contains your obligations and needs during the day. Some of these may overlap with wants:

- Work

- Exercise

- Healthy, wholesome diet

- Interaction with significant other and/or children and family

- Studies, if applicable

- Sleep

- Errands, such as cooking, groceries, cleaning and bills.

Based on this list, you may think it's impossible to have an accomplished day, and still have enough time for sleep. But keep reading and you will discover just how easy it is to balance everything.

●You work hours are already set. So, these give you set boundaries around which you can plan your day.

●Exercise is one of the most difficult activities to balance with your daily life. However, there are a few easy ways that you can fit exercise into a busy schedule. following these tips, you can fit exercise into your day without compromising your sleep cycle:

○Wake up earlier and go for a quick cardio and weight lifting session right before work.

○On some days, you may choose to sacrifice TV for exercise.

oWhenever you are idle, engage in exercise instead.

oWalk to work

oTry to incorporate exercise into other tasks. For example, if you are memorizing a speech, do so as you are exercising. Workout while you are watching TV. If you are struggling to make time for your significant other, go on a nice jog with them. That way, you can spend quality time and you can exercise simultaneously.

oTurn down unnecessary tasks.

oGo dancing with that special someone. Make exercise fun!

oYour chores can be your exercise.

oTake the stairs instead of the elevator.

•Eating healthy requires that you prepare healthy meals, or you purchase them outside of home. If you are interested in saving money, wake up early to prepare meals in advance. You can also do this before going to bed. On days that are especially busy, consider purchasing food, instead of cooking it. Otherwise, let your significant other take over cooking duties on occasion.

•Sometimes, when you have a busy schedule, you gradually spend less and less time with your family and spouse. Use this quality time as an incentive to work harder during the day. Otherwise, turn tasks into family activities. This may refer to exercising by playing outside with the kids or preparing healthy meals together as a family.

•If you are currently balancing studies with a job, decrease the amount of studying you have to do outside of the class by being totally immersed in class and extra attentive. Try to schedule a set time for all errands. Or, simply schedule automatic bill payments, or balance these responsibilities with someone else.

●**Sleep,** the purpose of this book. Once you have mastered the tips listed above, you will have more time to sleep. Ensure that you have an hour before bed to relax adequately and enter a sleep state.

Chapter 10: Classifications Of Sleep Apnea

There are 3 kinds of sleep apnea, yet just 2 are discussed the most. There is obstructive sleep apnea, which is the most frequent type for this condition. With obstructive sleep apnea, your throat muscles collapse as you're sleeping.

The other kind of sleep apnea is referred to as central sleep apnea. This type occurs when your breathing muscles do not get the appropriate signals. The third one, which many people do not experience, is called complex or mixed sleep apnea. This kind is a mix of both conditions.

Obstructive Sleep Apnea

Obstructive sleep apnea, or OSA, obstructs the air passage in your throat. Some other things that occur with this kind of sleep disorder are:

- As you're sleeping, the throat muscles collapse inward as you're breathing.

- Air is going to pass through the upper airway. This consists of the nose, mouth and throat areas.

- As the muscles get broader, they obstruct the collapse in order for the airway to stay open.

- You are going to have less oxygen in your blood. This induces your lungs to take in air from the outside.

- Apnea occurs when the back throat tissues are momentarily obstructed. You stop breathing, and if you wake up, you might need to gasp for breath.

- Even when you do gasp for air or make snoring sounds, you might not always get up.

In case you experience 5 or more apnea episodes per hour, it is considered to be part of obstructive sleep apnea.

Central Sleep Apnea

Central sleep apnea is not as frequent as obstructive sleep apnea. This kind of sleep apnea begins in the brain. The brain will not send a signal to the airway muscles so that they can breathe.

The level of oxygen declines, and you are going to most likely wake up. With this kind of sleep apnea, individuals typically remember waking up. If you have heart disease or cardiac arrest, then you are experiencing central sleep apnea.

Complex or Mixed Apnea

As pointed out previously, this is the mix of obstructive and central sleep apnea. With this kind of sleep apnea, you are going to deal with obstructive sleep apnea, or OSA. In addition to that, with good pressure from the airway, you are going to have continual central sleep apnea.

If you are utilizing CPAP (Continuous Positive Airway Pressure), the central sleep apnea is going to be acknowledged. This occurs after the obstruction has actually been cleared.

Chapter 11: Defining Insomnia

Doctors and health care experts refer to insomnia as a difficulty getting to sleep or staying asleep even if an individual has the time or opportunity to do so.Most individuals with episodes of insomnia feel displeased with the quality and amount of their sleep.Furthermore, they often experience difficulty in concentrating, fatigue, decreased performance at work/school, low energy and mood disturbances.

Insomnia may be characterized depending on the episode's duration in an individual.For instance, **acute insomnia** occurs briefly and is often caused by life events or circumstances such as receiving bad or stressful news or reviewing for an exam.This is the most common type of insomnia in which many people overcome without going through any treatment.

On the other hand, **chronic insomnia** occurs at least 3 nights every week and can last up to 3 months or more.It is disrupted sleep that is often caused by unhealthy sleeping habits, other types of medical conditions, changes in the environment, work shifts and some medications that result to insufficient sleep patterns.More often than not, chronic insomnia can be cured through various forms of treatment that help people acquire healthy sleep habits.Most cases of chronic insomnia are associated with another medical problem or mental disorder.

As mentioned earlier, individuals with insomnia are inclined to have difficulty falling asleep, staying asleep and even wake up too early than they should.The treatments for insomnia can include psychological, behavioral, medical methods or a combination of methods.

Although insomnia can be cured through medical treatments, there are also natural treatments available.For instance, if you want to have better sleep during the night, avoid drinking beverages with caffeine specifically in the later part of the day.You can also set regular times for waking up.It would also help to use thick blinds, curtains, earplugs or eye mask to avoid waking up due to light and noise especially in the middle of your sleep.Relaxation methods such as meditation, yoga, calming music or bathing with warm water can also help prepare for a good night's sleep.

Knowing If You Have Insomnia: The Symptoms

Prior to taking a step for any type of treatment, it is important to determine if you indeed have insomnia or just a passing sleep problem.Insomnia is usually chronic specifically if the difficulty in falling or staying asleep transpires at least thrice a week for three months or more.Most people may have experienced short periods of insomnia at one point of their lives.Thus, it can be quite tricky to determine if you have a more severe form of insomnia that necessitates treatment or just a normal, temporary sleep problem.

On the other hand, you would be able to discern the type of sleep problem if you know the symptoms of insomnia.Based on several studies, an individual with insomnia may have one or more insomnia symptom.These may include difficulty in getting to sleep; difficulty in staying asleep or returning to sleep; has low energy or fatigue; waking up too early than necessary; has non-restorative sleep; cognitive impairment including concentration difficulty; behavior problems including aggression or feeling impulsive; mood disturbance including irritability; difficulty in personal relationships; and/or difficulty at work/school.

When discerning if you have insomnia or just a passing sleep problem, it is important to take note of the duration of the episode.Your episode may be considered chronic insomnia if it transpires at least 3 times a week for 3 months or more.If this is the case, your insomnia may be considered either a behavioral pattern or comorbid, which means it is associated with another medical issue that needs treatment.Chronic insomnia can be characterized as a behavioral pattern if your schedule of sleep is not synced with your body clock or your routines/activities during the night do not prepare your body for sleep.

Based on recent studies, insomnia is being thought as a problem in which the brain is unable to stop being awake.The brain involves sleep and wake cycles.If the sleep cycle is on, the wake cycle is off and vice versa.Thus, insomnia can be a disorder with either of the cycles wherein there is too little sleep drive or too much wake drive.Irrespective of the cause of insomnia once it transpires on a regular basis, it is best to consult your doctor to address the problem at once.

It is also advisable to determine how insomnia affects your life.For instance, if you wake up feeling tired or having low energy and this continues throughout the day, it may affect your productivity at work/school as well as your activities with family and friends.If you tried to address the issue on your own and failed, this could mean you need to consult your doctor to prevent more serious problems.

Chapter 12: Natural Ways To Aid Sleep

Meditation and relaxation techniques

Your stress levels can affect your sleep and it can be difficult to lower them. Using meditation and other relaxation techniques can slow your breathing and direct your attention to an object of focus. When your mind is filled with outside stimuli it can be hard to relax. These techniques will help you concentrate and increase awareness.

● **Visualization**: Involve all your senses and imagine a place that relaxes you. Think of a beach with the sea lapping at the shores and the feel of sunshine on your bare skin. You can hear the waves, smell the sea and feel the warm breeze on your skin. Imagine lying back on a towel and closing your eyes. Drift off to the sound of the ocean and the warmth of the summer sun.

- **Mindfulness**: Focus on the positive aspects of your life and what you can do to improve them. Appreciate all the great connections you have with your family and friend and thank the universe for the joy in your life.

- **7-11 breathing technique**: This technique is designed to regulate your breathing and prepare you for sleep. Breathe in for 7 seconds and then breathe out for 11 seconds. Lay in your favorite position and repeat until you fall asleep. The constant counting will help you focus on your mind, muscles, and body and help them relax.

- **Squeeze and relax:** As you are lying in bed focus on one group of muscles at a time. Squeeze them until tense and then relax them. Your mind will be calmed by the actions and your body will relax.

Herbal Sleep Aids

The herb Vitex Agnus Castus - also known as chaste tree - can help cure insomnia during menstruation. Studies have shown that women suffering from PMS can benefit from taking the chaste tree. However, this herb should not be taken when on birth control pills, hormone replacement therapy or any dopamine-based medication.

Valerian is an herbal home-brewed remedy that can provide relief from insomnia and aid sleep. A standard dose of 450mg should be taken an hour before bedtime and should be taken with food.

Valerian is thought to increase the levels of calming neutron transmitters in the body and can relieve muscle spasms.

Lemon balm is available as a supplement or in tea form and is said to relieve anxiety and calm the nervous system. Sleep aid supplements with lemon balm generally contain valerian as well.

General hacks for a better sleep

• No pets: This can be a tough one for some people, but you can't expect a good night's sleep when you have your fluffy companions in your bed. Studies have shown that you are 63% more likely to have a poor night's sleep if your pets are with you.

• Sleep on the left side of your body: Experts recommend sleeping on your left as it improves your circulation and combats heartburn and acid reflux. You are also less likely to be interrupted.

● Don't look at the clock: Sneaking a peek at the clock to see how long it is before you wake up will only cause you anxiety.

● Don't leave things undone: Doing the washing up and other unpleasant tasks before you go to bed will help you relax. If you are worried about paying the bills or general household tasks you will be less likely to relax.

● Take a cold bath: We all know the benefits of a warm bath but can a cold dip before bedtime do you good? Experts have proved that a cold bath an hour before sleep can help lower the temperatures of the body. This helps the process of falling to sleep and is like being hit with a tranquilizer.

• Allow your feet freedom: When you are dreaming or having a nightmare you will often imagine running or moving your feet. If your bedclothes are restricting your feet you will feel anxious and this can wake you up even when you are experiencing deep sleep.

Have you considered the position you sleep in? There are studies that show instinctive sleeping patterns that nomads and forest dwellers adapt can help with musculoskeletal health and help correct joint pain.

Mountain gorillas naturally sleep on one side and use a laterally rotated arm as a pillow. Native Kenyans adopt the same position that allows them to listen for danger with both ears.

Tibetan caravanners have been pictured sleeping on their shins. This position may seem unnatural for the "civilized" world, but nature tells us differently. The anterior border of the tibia and the medial border of the ulna are the only parts of the body that are in contact with the ground when sleeping in this position. This minimizes the loss of heat while the folded position of the body also conserves heat. The position also allows the sleeper to have both ears alert for any foe and prevents them from revealing their position by making a noise. As the head is facing down this closes the mouth and makes it impossible to snore.

Of course, we are not suggesting you abandon your pillows and sleep like a gorilla or indeed a Tibetan caravanner, but a change of position might make all the difference. Try sleeping in the military crawl position and limit the movement of your body during sleep. Lie face down on your bed and tilt your head to expose your right cheek. Lift your right arm into a crooked position so it points above your head. Your right leg should be bent at the knee and face outward at an angle to your stomach.

Imagine a soldier crawling under a net and replicate the position. Some cultures use this position to prevent babies and younger children from moving when they need to be calm. Less movement means faster sleep.

Final note: Some people are just not meant to sleep in the same bed. We may love the idea of spooning with our partners until we both drift off into a romantic sleep and waking in a mutual embrace. The reality is that your partner may snore, pass wind or just take all the bedding. If you find you are losing sleep because of your partner, consider sleeping in different beds. Different schedules and even different temperature preferences can cause a loss of sleep. You may even find yourself enjoying the time you do spend together in the bedroom more knowing that you are going to sleep well after! Remember the two things the bedroom is for? Why not improve both?

Chapter 13: Limit Use Of Electronic Devices Before Bed

Technological gadgets have become too much a part of our lives. We have become so dependent and attached to them that we can almost not live without them. We are constantly looking at our phones, tablets, laptops, TVs, playing video games and others. These devices are useful as they enable us to connect with the world but they are also somewhat of a disruption when it comes to sleep. It's a common thing for many people to check on their devices when they are in bed, chat with a few friends, read an email or even play a video game. You'll even fall asleep as you hold your phone and wake up later at night to check on something. These electronics are eating the time we should be sleeping thus preventing us from getting a good night's sleep. This is not the only effect they have on our sleep.

These devices emit light on their screens. This light will affect the production of melatonin which is the sleep inducing hormone. With lower melatonin, we are unable to sleep and when we manage to, we have interruptions due to poor transition between cycles. These devices emit the blue wavelength light which is received by photoreceptors in the retina. They mislead the brain on the status of the day. The brain needs to get ready for sleep. You just don't lie in bed and close your eyes to fall asleep. Children and adolescents are most affected by this blue light from electronic devices. A study carried out on children who used various devices before sleeping found out that they had concentration problems during the day which was attributed to a lower quality of sleep as compared to their counterparts. They also slept for fewer hours thus failing to fulfill their sleep requirements. Experts advise that you should not use any gadget an hour before sleep. This may sound almost impossible but remember what we discovered in the last chapter, if you prioritize sleep, you'll do anything to have a quality night's sleep. Finish up on all your activities that require a device well in advance, not unless it's an emergency. To this end, get all gadgets out of the bedroom, most especially TV sets and laptops. Don't even go with your phone to the bedroom.

Another reason why we shouldn't be using our gadgets before sleep is because they stimulate the brain and make it remain active while we should be preparing to sleep. For instance, if you work on some emails, play a video game, watch a movie or engage in a long conversation on your phone right before you sleep, you engage the brain and make it active. Now before you sleep, the brain has to unwind and transition from an active state to an idle state for you to fall asleep.

Another reason to get rid of all electronic devices from the bedroom is the fact that these devices will interrupt sleep by their ringing and vibration. You notice how our brain is very sensitive to our usual ringtone such that even when in deep sleep, you are likely to wake up when this sound is played. You may even not consciously realize it but your sleep will be interfered with. Our goal here is to have a good night's sleep, not just the amount of hours we spend in bed. So remove all these gadgets from the bedroom.

According to experts, children, adolescents and even adults have formed a habit of having their hand held devices when in bed as an opportunity to catch up with friends on social media platforms. This learned association is quite unhealthy. The bed is primarily for sleeping and associating it with any other activity will affect the quality of sleep.

Chapter 14: 3 Things To Do Before You Go To Sleep

A large portion of us have a tendency to have a short agenda of things that we have to do before we rest around evening time. These incorporate such things as ensuring that the sink is clear of any dishes, forgetting the mutts and verifying whether the entryways are bolted. On the off chance that we are managing sleep deprivation, in any case, we should ensure that we have an agenda of things to do with a specific end goal to cure this normally too. Here are three unique things that we ought to do each night with a specific end goal to help us to get some profound rest before the time has come to wake up once more.

The primary thing that you ought to do is to ensure that your condition is spotless. This is not just valid for your territory where you will be resting, it is additionally valid for your body. Despite the fact that we are not going to have the capacity to see the way that our room is perfect at whatever point we are dozing, our brain will realize that it is. An uncluttered situation will unclutter your psyche and enable you to rest unhampered amid the night. Ensuring that your body is spotless will likewise enable you to get a decent evenings to rest. One reason why this is the situation is on the grounds that dust tends to gather in our hair amid the day. On the off chance that hypersensitivities are an issue, washing your hair will expel this wellspring of unfavorably susceptible responses.

The second thing that you ought to do each night is to set up your brain for a decent evenings rest. Try not to enable anything to fortify you rationally inside the quick hour before you rest. This would incorporate the things that you watch on TV and additionally the things that you may read. Focus on unwinding things and enable your psyche to float to quieting contemplations. This will go far in helping you to rest throughout the night.

At last, you should ensure that your whole family unit is set up for you to rest legitimately. The two greatest rest executioners are commotion and light. Ensure that everyone comprehends that you require things to be calm with the goal for you to rest soundly. You ought to likewise consider putting resources into a few blinds or maybe an eye cover with the goal for it to be as dim as could reasonably be expected. Both of these things will help you to nod off rapidly and to stay unconscious as long as possible.

Chapter 15: Spirit, Restore Your Soul And Restore Your Sleep

Again, I want to remind you that when I talk about restoring your spirit and spirituality in general I am not talking about religious beliefs or any particular religion at all. Whatever makes you feel at peace, whatever makes you feel connected, open and comfortable is what you should consider as your spirituality. Please feel free to adapt and change things to suit your personal tastes and your religious foundation as you see fit.

I would like for you to think back to a time when you felt guilty about something. Maybe it was something that you think you could have done differently. Perhaps you missed an opportunity to help out a friend or family member. Maybe you told a lie to a loved one. Now, how did you sleep that night? Did you toss and turn? Did you stare at the ceiling until the wee hours of the morning? If you slept at all did you have terrible dreams that eventually woke you, sweaty and upset? What did you do then? Did you apologize or try to make amends in some small way? Did that help your sleeping?

The spirit is often the part of your care that is so often overlooked and under-nourished. We eat good foods because we want good health. We read and learn new things because we want an active and functional brain but what do we do about our spiritual health? You will almost never hear a doctor suggest that you meditate or pray or volunteer at the local dog shelter in hopes of reconnecting with your spiritual side but why not?

Studies have confirmed the benefit of prayer on health. Additional studies have confirmed that meditation, yoga and even just walking barefoot allow for a reconnection to the spiritual as well as to the Earth, literally grounding a person. Still, people seem to be reluctant to accept that something as simple as saying a prayer or repeating a soothing mantra or even just thinking of a beautiful sunset can help them in any way, let alone to get more sleep.

Sleep itself is often considered spiritual in a way. For some people dreams can be a way of receiving the messages that Nature or a Higher Power wants them to have- the same messages that they are just too busy to hear during the day. Some people say they never remember their dreams or can only remember bits and pieces of it. Others remember every detail of their dream with amazing clarity. And then there are the true Dream Masters- the people who can not only remember their dreams but can control much of the action of the dream while they are sleeping. Sometimes called "lucid dreaming", these people have evolved into a state of conscious but not conscious thinking that allows them to set the stage, control the action and the direction of the dream and even change the outcome if they want. These people frequently are very good at sleeping, usually because they want to get back to the dream they left the night before.

For the rest of us, there are ways to reconnect with the spirit and get back to better and more restful sleep. First, define what spirituality means to you. It is important to make this connection as much about your own personal code and belief system as possible. Once you have defined that, you will go on to defining what enhances, what helps and what moves your spirit the most. Some people get tripped up on this part because they think that doing things to help the spirit must be purely altruistic and they are stumped as to what they can do-everything that they think of gives them benefits as well. That is perfectly fine, in fact, that is the point. You want to flood your spirit with those positive feelings so that you have something to reflect on. That night, when you get ready for bed you can say to yourself "Look what I have done today" and you should feel satisfied, proud of yourself but most importantly, ready to sleep.

Here are some suggestions and exercises for reconnecting to your spiritual side:

Exercise One:Try Meditation

For some people, the simple act of sitting still for any period of time is nearly impossible. For some reason, everyone is convinced that they must be on the go, go, go all of the time. No wonder we cannot sleep! Meditation is not just about sitting still, however. It is about learning to focus your brain and your awareness, about learning to control not only your thoughts but your breathing as well. You must learn to be able to shut out negative thoughts. You have to be able to shut out the environment you are sitting in.

How you choose to meditate is up to you. Some people choose to sit on the ground; some prefer a cushion or even a chair. Your comfort is very important especially as you are learning the practice. A focal point can be very helpful and can be something as simple as a candle flame. If you are comfortable with silence, this is fine but if not, gentle and rhythmic music can help to set a pattern for your breathing and your heart rate. Some people are most happy with a guided meditation, which is simply a CD or DVD that takes you through the imagery and the breathing for the practice. Set a short goal for yourself, say five minutes and then work your way up to longer and longer practices.

Exercise Two:Try Restorative Yoga

There are many yoga poses (pranas) that are specifically meant to improve sleep and restfulness. To that end, there are a great many full practices that are meant to be restful and relaxing. As previously mentioned, some people are not comfortable with even yoga close to their bedtime so if that is you, please skip this suggestion. If you do choose to try yoga remember these things: there is no such thing as the "perfect" yoga pose. Yoga is about achieving something in the moment, not competing or comparing. You will find that you are flexible one day and stiffer the next. Always adjust each pose to how you are feeling that particular day and never push beyond what you are ready for. Focus on breathing. If you are following a practice on DVD or audio, listen to the cuing and allow yourself to surrender to the poses.

A few poses to get you started include Child's Pose, which is often referred to as "mouse pose", Reclined Bound Angle Pose and Legs up the Wall Pose.

If you would prefer to follow a DVD, I would recommend Rodney Yee who has some very gentle, relaxing practices that are perfect for beginners. Yee has a pleasant and welcoming demeanor as well as a very relaxing voice.

Exercise Three:Start a Dream Journal

When you wake up in the morning, focus on what you remember from your dreams and then write them down. How did you feel about the dream? Who was in them? What were they doing? Try to be as detailed as possible when you are writing in your dream journal. Let this be a way to reconnect with what your spirit and your subconscious self is trying to tell you. Next, see if you can guide your dreams at all. Write in the dream journal what you would like to dream about the following night and then see how well you did.

Exercise Four: The Everyday Samaritan

Every day find something, even as simple as complimenting a stranger or holding a door for someone and then do it. Some days you may be able to do something bigger. One day you might have an extra few minutes and you can round up all of the carts in the supermarket parking lot so that the employees do not have to come out to do it. Or, you have an extra five in your pocket so you hand it to the drive-thru employee for the car behind you. You know that you made a stranger smile. They don't know who you are and hopefully they will do the same for someone when they are able. Volunteer to walk and socialize the dogs at the animal shelter. Take part in a charity fun run (or volunteer at one if running is not your thing). Just find something and then do it. The point is to have something to look back on and be proud of yourself.

Exercise Five:Reconnect with Nature

Finally, too many people spend all of their time inside of their homes and inside of their office buildings and not enough time in nature. Go to a park or to the beach and stare at the trees and the water. Hike a nature trail. Walk barefoot in the grass. Reestablishing a connection to nature and the Earth can also reset your inner clock, the one that helps you know when to fall asleep and when to wake up.

Chapter 16: Breathing Exercises To Help You Sleep Better

Over the years, studies have shown that being kind to yourself makes you happy, which allows you to get better quality rest. With this in mind, it is important to visualize your pleasant experiences, so that the mind and heart absorbs them and brings about positive change. This can be achieved by practicing breathing exercises. There are many simple ways to embed positive experiences into the psyche. We're going to focus on a diaphragmatic breathing exercise to help improve your quality of sleep.

What is Diaphragmatic breathing? This is a method that helps you use the diaphragm to breathe correctly. Besides improving the quality of sleep, this has many benefits.

It improves oxygen flow to your brain

It strengthens your diaphragm

It's less effort and energy while you breathe

Let's get started on this technique:

Lie down on your back on a flat surface and get in a comfortable position. You can use a pillow for your head and another one to place under your knees. Place one of your hands at the top of your chest and the other in the middle of your stomach.

Start by breathing in slowly through your nose and make sure you focus on all the air coming into your diaphragm first before breathing any air into your chest. If you do this correctly, you will start to feel your stomach move out, and should not have any movement from your hand at the top of your chest.

After you've taken a deep breath through your nose and filled your diaphragm with air, breathe in more air in through your chest. It will feel a little weird because you might start to feel a bit light-headed, but this is normal, and this actually helps get more oxygen to your brain, which is a good thing.

Try taking about 10-15 of these deep breaths for starters. You should feel a lot more relaxed after doing this exercise. This is actually a great breathing technique that will relax you, and if you get good at it, you can use it anytime for stress relief too.

If you plan to perform this exercise while sitting in a chair, the technique will be the same except you will be sitting upright in a chair.

Practice this technique for about 5-10 minutes, and 2-3 times a day. It will become easier and easier the more you practice it.

Chapter 17: Lifestyle And Behavioral Treatments

It has been mentioned several times in the previous chapters that modifications in your lifestyle habits might do the trick in treating your sleep disorders and sleeping problems. Listed here is what doctors call lifestyle and behavioral treatments to help you sleep better.

Stimulus Control – The bedroom should always promote sleep and relaxation. Television sets and entertainment systems have no place in the bedroom.

Sleep Restriction Therapy – Doctors recommend that you should get up the moment you wake up and lay in bed only to sleep. Prolonged stay in bed other than to sleep only worsens the symptoms.

145

Cognitive Therapy – This is used to treat insomnia. The treatment includes the proper identification of the root cause of the disorder. It gives information to patients about age-related sleep changes, sleep norms, and the impact of taking naps and of being physically active on having a good night's sleep.

Relaxation Training – Several methods are taught to patients, like the PMR or Progressive Muscle Relaxation technique. PMR aims to help patients to relax the major muscle groups. Other techniques are imagery, self-hypnosis, and deep breathing techniques. Patients are asked to practice relaxation training techniques on a daily basis to ensure success.

Sleep Hygiene – This takes into consideration the following factors: your habits, common sleep practices, and environment influences. The four general areas that sleep hygiene concentrates on are your age, internal biological clock, psychological stressors causing difficulty in sleeping, and substances like caffeine, nicotine, and alcohol.

Your sleep patterns usually change when you turn 40. As people age, nocturnal awakenings become more frequent. These awakenings can affect the quality of sleep you get.
Your internal biological clock or the circadian rhythm determines how much sleep you get.

Psychological stressors include job-related deadlines or exams and schoolwork that cause you to lose sleep at night. Most people tend to worry about the next day's activities even when they are about to sleep, causing them to lay awake for hours which then results in inadequate sleep.

When you drink caffeinated drinks before bedtime, you might not be able to doze off right away. Nicotine also has the same effect. While alcohol has a sedating effect, thus making you sleep immediately, it is quickly metabolized as you sleep, causing arousals in the middle of the night. The sleeping environment should promote sleep. It has to be cool, silent, and with very little to no light at all. Patients are often advised to put up heavy curtains and wear earplugs and eye covers.

Chapter 18: Still Awake?! Let's Count...

If all, or most of the above do not put you to sleep, you might find yourself staring at the ceiling and doubting your own investment in the mattress. Is it the new pajamas? Why is the music and the aromatherapy not working for you? Your mind might be telling you that it is time to start counting sheep, which is the cheapest and a time-proven way to help you sleep. Reality check, it has never worked for me. Counting sheep, or any other farm, desert or zoo animal! Though there are a few "counting" exercises that can really help your mind relax and zone out.

Prepare a to-do list. Have a notepad next to your bed and start scribbling down a list of things to do during the next day or week. Not only will it help you have a list of things ready in the morning, but it will also help your mind to find order and sense in the middle of random thoughts. Sometimes we are kept awake because our unconscious mind is thinking of something that you really need to do, but may have forgotten. Well, bring it all out and put it in the notepad, it will bring peace to your mind.

Count your blessings. Be thankful for what you have and do not worry about what you do not have. Sometimes it's those thoughts that keep you awake, always wondering about all the negative events in your life or all the negativity from family or friends. Turn your mind to positive thoughts. Keep pictures on your wall from a family vacation that will bring you happy thoughts or even framed awards from your work, competitive events or any other achievements.

Count from 1 to 7 as you breathe. Breathing exercises are great to help you fall asleep, coupled with meditation techniques. These will help you focus your mind and clear your thoughts. There are a lot of ways to do it, but basically, they all come down to counting upwards to 7 as you inhale slowly and then downwards back to 1 as you exhale. Keep doing it and focus your mind on a specific thought or a positive word that you like. Allow your mind to go deeper into yourself and forget about your struggles with sleep.

Get up from the bed and go outside, count the stars. I do this a lot when everything else fails. I just get out from the bed and take a walk. Look up to the sky and let my mind drift into thoughts of infinity, space walks, and aliens. Once my imagination is going, it makes it so much easier to go back into the room and start dreaming.

Chapter 19: Who Is At Risk For Sleep Apnea?

Anybody, at any age can suffer from Sleep Apnea. However, there is a typical trend that has been noticed among people with Sleep Apnea. It has been observed that people belonging to a particular race, age or even gender can be impacted more than the rest of the population. See below;

Gender

Men are more prone to develop Sleep Apnea than women. Sleep Apnea can also be linked with excessive daytime sleeping, which is more common in men than women. Studies have consistently shown that men experience Sleep Apnea symptoms more as compared to the women.

153

Sex differences are also linked with the pathological difference between a man and a woman. The anatomical frame of the upper airway differs in males and females. The upper airway is typically larger in men than that of women.

Magnetic resonance is used to determine the sex related variances in the upper airway of men and women. Similarly, the size of the soft neck tissues is found to be greater in men. All these pathological differences result in more Sleep Apnea related issues in men.

Age

There is a good chance that the older you get, the more susceptible you become to Sleep Apnea. People can suffer from Sleep Apnea at any age, but as you get older, you become more susceptible due to the aging process. Softening of the skin and tissue in the throat can result in Sleep Apnea problems above the age of 45.

Genetics

The link between genetic problems and Sleep Apnea cannot be ignored. Families where one or more members have suffered from Sleep Apnea are likely to pass on this condition to the future generations.

It is possible if any one of your parents, grandparents or siblings once suffered from this disorder, you may also be prone to it. Such genetic problems can only be detected through DNA marking tests that could educate you about all the possible conditions you can suffer from. Such tests, if conducted early, can be immensely helpful in steering clear of various ailments.

Excessive alcohol consumption

Some people believe that alcohol can act as a muscle relaxant and treat their Apnea issues. However, studies say otherwise. In fact, if you are experiencing sleep problems, alcohol consumption can make it worse.

Considering alcohol being a muscle relaxant, people with Sleep Apnea tend to slow down or stop breathing for longer spans. Excessive alcohol can also interfere with REM sleep, which is needed for proper functioning of the brain or memory. Excessive sweating and/or extreme anxiety or sleepiness in the daytime due to alcohol can only worsen your problems at hand.

Race

It is true that people belonging to different races have different instances of Sleep Apnea. A particular study has implied that not only age groups, but even the race of a person determines whether he/she is likely to suffer from Sleep Apnea or not. African-Americans have been found more prone to develop Sleep Apnea problems than Caucasians, Hispanic or Asian ethnicity.

Chapter 20: Natural Healing

As with all ailments and abnormal processes that affect the body, one of the best ways to recover from an abnormal issue is to return to nature. Before you can consider this, you must pose two questions and answer this truthfully. The first is about your general lifestyle. Have you engaged in a lifestyle that is far from the way the body was intended? In many cases, this answer is in the affirmative.

The second is concerned with your will to recover from this. If you are strong to undergo the changes, then you will be able to experience a total recovery. If you are not committed then the best route for you is the surgical and pharmaceutical route.

We will assume you have answered in the affirmative to both questions.

The first thing you need to do to experience the benefits of a natural healing, is to return your lifestyle to the way you r body intended it. There are too many forces at work for you to try and figure out which is causing the breathing disorder. Just as it will be difficult to diagnose the ensuing kidney failure or the heart failure that comes from tired muscles when there is diminished oxygen flowing to the major muscle groups. The only way to do it is allow the body to return itself to optimal condition and doing this requires the return to nature.

The first step in returning to nature requires that you return to a vegetarian diet. There are other things you need to do if you are a vegetarian. However, for those of you who consume meat, the first step is to exclude all meat, poultry and aquatic food.

By converting to vegetarianism, you begin to reduce the toxins that are inherent in processed meats and meat in general. Remember the problem with meat is not just that it is meat, but also because of what the animal is fed in captivity. The toxin build up is slow and over time it begins to affect various symptoms and one of those that are effected are the airways and the toxicity in the brainstem.

The first step is to slowly cut out the meats and increase the intake of green vegetables, pulses, beans, fruits and nuts as well as seeds. The human body is designed to consume food that can be digested slowly and food where, once digested, the nutrients can be extracted over time. It is not designed to consume food that turns putrid rapidly, as in the case of meet. When you compare the length of the digestive tract of a lion and man, you will see that the true carnivore has a short tract to allow the meats to exit the body before it putrefies. In cows, on the other hand, they have four stomachs to keep digesting the grass they eat and they have long tracts to absorb the nutrients.

Man's digestive tract is relatively long and undigested meat can sometimes be stuck and putrefy, releasing toxins into the blood stream that can penetrate the brain stem and disrupt its regular operation. Removal of these toxins is of the highest importance especially when you are looking to heal nervous system issues.

Once you have turned to vegetarianism, the next step is to detox your body from the putrefying contents of you gut. To do this, start with a fruit diet and psyllium husk. If you are allergic to psyllium husk, increase the fiber content in your food while you are on the fruit diet.

During the fruit diet phase, which must prolong for three days, you will need to eat the fruits whole, do not juice them. If you juice them, add a teaspoon of psyllium husk and drink that, but limit that to only once a day. At other times, eat a variety of fruits and drink mineral water with lemon juice squeezed in. This helps to balance your blood's pH.

At the end of three days, monitor your bowel movements and the consistence and color of the product. What you are looking for is long, soft and do not be surprised if the odor is highly offensive. That just means the three-day fruit diet is working. The putrefying matter is exiting your system.

Once you complete the first three days, return to a vegetarian diet that is low in salt and sugar. Go online and find a list of vegetarian items that are not acidic and combine those with nuts and seeds as well as herbs and spices.Stay away from the nightshade variety of vegetables. These are highly acidic and will wreak havoc with your system.

A week after you start your diet, start your next water diet. At this point, you will only consume mineral water for three full days. There will be no solid food and no supplements. At the end of the three days, break fast with ripe mangoes. Followed by any fruit your body tells you.

A week after that, meaning two weeks from the day you started the fruit fast, you will start the next three-day water fast. This will be your third week and your second water fast.

On your fourth week, you will begin a one-week fast. If you have the ability to check in to a fast farm or do this under professional supervision, it would be better. If not, do this under the supervision of a family member or friend. Fast for one week and consume nothing but water.

At the end of four weeks, you would have lost some weight and you will notice that any signs of OSA would have abated. However, if you are suffering from CSA you will still need to do more. CSA is a serious condition because it is indicating that there is something seriously wrong with your CNS or the nerves that form the signalling chain. There is no other way to repair this than to get your body to do it.

If you have CNS, you need to check into a fast camp and commit to a three-week fast. This three-week fast will allow you to fix everything in your own body. When your body is not busy digesting food, it will begin the process of healing.

The biggest benefit of a three-week fast is that the body will go though a number of stages. In the first stage, the body will shift metabolic pathways. This just means that it changes its source of energy from what is in the gut to what is in the fat cells. Once the body changes to absorb energy from the fat cells, it will consume all the fat over the course of the fast and the body will stop feeling hungry. However, the mind will continue to invoke the sense of hunger because of habit. At this point, it's a matter of controlling your mind. You are not starving.

Starving is a point when your body is not able to find fat tissue to convert o energy and it starts to consume the protein in muscles. On the other hand, fasting happens once all the food in the gut is consumed and the body goes after the fat.

Between the point of fasting and starvation, there is one intermediate point where the body goes after alien tissue and consumes it for energy. There have even been claims of people curing cancer in this way, as the body starts to consume the cancer cells. The body also starts to heal scars and growths. People even report better eyesight, better hearing and even better sense of smell. A renewal returns the body to almost brand new.

The three-week time limit for the fast is an average length. The true determinant on when to break the fast is based on how your body feels. A person who is large and has a lot of fat tissue can obviously last a lot longer than three weeks, while a person with zero fat will not be able to last as long. The key to knowing when to break the fast is to listen to your body.

The signal is simple. Your body will start to feel a deep and intense hunger, and that will be your signal to break fast. When you do, start with water, followed by mangoes and yoghurt. That's it. Do not eat anything else. You need to repopulate your digestive tract with good bacteria and yoghurt is a good way to do that. The following day, have more fruits and more yoghurt and introduce easily digestive vegetables sautéed in clarified butter (ghee). Do not add salt or sugar to your cooking. In fact, this is a good time for you to throw out all sugar and salt from your pantry - you do not need them anymore. Your taste buds will be able to relish the natural taste of food.

On the third day, still include yoghurt, but you can now start consuming a number of other vegetables, puree them in the blender and consume small quantities at a time. You will notice that it takes very little to get you satisfied. Your body has become highly efficient in sourcing for what it needs. It will take a couple of days before you get a regular bowel movement and when you do, you will notice no smell and your urine will also be clear and odorless.

By this point in time, if you have done everything right, your sleep apnea will be gone. There will be not obstructions, and your CNS will be functioning correctly again. You will find that you sleep more effectively and you will awake before the alarm clock and before the sun rises.

Chapter 21: Creating A Sanctuary

Room Function: Treat the bedroom as a room that is exclusively for sleeping. When the brain associates a specific room with the act of sleeping, it will automatically trigger the necessary preparations for sleep. A bedroom should be a sanctuary that promotes relaxation. Ideally, it should have a restful and stress-relieving environment.

Sleep Solution Tips:

Avoid incorporating a work area into the space to maintain the primary function of the bedroom.

Keep television sets, computers, and other potentially distracting items out of the bedroom.

A humidifier can help to improve the quality of the air and help to improve the quality of sleep as well.

Plants are a great way of keeping the bedroom air from being stale.

Studies show that Jasmine can help to improve a person's quality of sleep.

Heat and Cold: Body temperatures figure greatly in the universal ability to sleep. A process called thermoregulation influences the cycles of sleep. To initiate sleep, the body's core temperature drops in preparation for a restive state. If the room temperature is too high, the body has a harder time keeping the ideal temperature that is adequate for sleep. Studies have shown that the best temperature at bedtime is about 60 to 68 degrees Fahrenheit. Temperatures above or below the given range can cause difficulties in sleeping.

Sleep Solution Tips:

Keep the bedroom temperature as close to the recommended range as possible.

Taking a warm bath or shower two hours before bedtime can help to lower down the body's core temperature.

Opening a window can help to keep air currents flowing for a cooler environment.

Running Water: Some people find that the sound of running water helps them relax and sleep better. Studies say that this is because the body's heartbeat and breathing slows down when a person listens to the said sound.

Sleep Solution Tip:

A table-top fountain or a mini waterfall can simulate running water and give off the desired sound.

Sleeping with a Partner: A lot of people have trouble sleeping next to someone else due to various reasons: too much body heat, snoring, limited sleep space, etc.

Sleep Solution Tips:

Consider having separate bedrooms or a separate bed away from your partner if you are feeling sleep deprived.

Keep pets out of the bedroom to avoid sleep disruption from them.

If you have a baby, consider putting him or her in a crib or in a separate nursery.

Ife separate bedrooms or beds are not an option, try to use separate blankets instead.

Noise Pollution: Most people find it difficult to fall asleep in a noisy environment. Noise pollution is often caused by outside noises such as: barking dogs or animal sounds, loud neighbors, and automobile or traffic sounds.

Sleep Solution Tips:

Consider wearing ear plugs to keep out external sounds.

Try masking sounds with a fan, recordings of soothing sounds, or white noise.

Wall Color and Theme: Studies show that certain colors stimulate different responses in the brain. Cool colors are often associated with tranquility and feelings of calm and peace. Most interior design experts recommend a light lilac shade on the walls of the bedroom to help reinforce a feeling or relaxation.

Linens, Pillows, Mattresses, and Blankets: What you sleep on is just as important as where you sleep. Comfort is the key when trying to get to that ideal state that puts you in a mood to rest. While some people prefer soft beddings, others might like firmer mattresses or pillows. Depending on your comfort levels, adjust things accordingly. Keeping everything fresh and clean may also help to induce sleep more easily. The right size of pillows is essential in getting a person comfortable enough throughout the whole duration of the sleep cycle.

Chapter 22: Indulge In Quality Evening "Me"Time

Do you have a special nighttime routine, or would you describe the things you do in the evenings as erratic? One of the reasons why some people fall asleep easily is their nighttime routines, and if you do not have a fixed one yourself, then it is high time to start.

Let's face it: human beings are creatures of habit. When we start to do something repeatedly, the action eventually becomes so deeply ingrained into the mind that it becomes automatic. This transition lasts for at least 21 days. In other words, do something for 21 consecutive days and it will become a habit.

Now it goes without saying that there are certain habits you may have during the evenings that are keeping you from falling asleep. On the bright side, you can replace these bad habits with ones that will actually **help** you fall asleep.

Once you combine these good habits into one cohesive system in the evening, you can increase your chances of getting great quality sleep naturally.

What are these nighttime habits that will help you fall asleep naturally? The best ones are explained in detail below:

Set your"go to bed"alarm.

If you are still building the habit of going to bed at the same time each night, then a gentle reminder will help you stay on track. If it takes you 15 minutes to fall asleep after getting to bed, and if you have to be asleep by 10:30 p.m. for instance, then you need to set this alarm to 10:15 p.m.

Eat a light dinner.

As explained Chapter 3, a light dinner, which consists of healthy natural foods will keep you from feeling hungry later on in the night. Ideally, you should eat your dinner no less than three hours before bedtime.

Take a warm bath or shower.

Cleansing your body with warm water will not only make you feel fresh, clean and ready for bed, but it will also help you relax. It would be even better to choose hygiene products with warm, relaxing scents such as lavender or jasmine. Try to avoid anything citrus or minty, as these are meant to energize you (best to reserve them for your morning showers, instead).

To maximize the sleep-inducing effects of a warm bath, you should then go stay in a room with the thermostat set to a cool temperature. Just make sure to bundle up so that you will not feel chilly.

Have a light snack or drink something warm and comforting.

If you are feeling just a little bit hungry before bedtime, you should nibble on any of the sleep-inducing snacks listed in Chapter 3. However, if you would rather have a nice, warm beverage, then a cup of warm milk or hot herbal tea will satisfy you all the same.

Brush your teeth and cleanse your face.

You may think it is ridiculous to be reminded to brush your teeth before bedtime, but you will be surprised at how people keep putting this off until late into the night. The reason why you should brush your teeth as soon as you have finished eating your final meal for the night is this: it will actually cue your brain that it is ready for bed.

The same idea applies to cleansing your face, especially to women who wear makeup every day. The simple habit of wiping off your makeup and putting on whatever evening moisturizers and toners you like will also signal you for sleep.

Plan and prepare for tomorrow.

This is a crucial habit to keep, especially if you are someone who constantly stays up late because of nagging thoughts about your responsibilities for tomorrow. It only takes a few minutes to plan ahead, but it will save you several hours from tossing and turning in bed later on. Here are simple strategies to help you build this habit:

Create a to-do list for tomorrow. A to-do list is one of the easiest ways to plan ahead. Anything that you need to accomplish should be jotted down. After that, tell yourself to not think about these tasks anymore. You have them on paper, so you should not worry about forgetting them. Nothing is worth sacrificing good quality sleep.

Choose your outfit for tomorrow. Also, consider assembling tomorrow's outfit in a specific spot. For example, you can choose what to wear for work tomorrow, then lay them on a chair. Doing so will save you a lot of time and effort in making decisions the next day.

Gather your things into one container. Aside from your clothes, put together all the things you need in a bag, suitcase, or tray. If you have important documents or other items that you must bring with you, place them in your bag that very night.

Shut down digital devices (or put them on airplane mode).

Stimulation from devices such as your smartphone, computer, and television, will keep your brain from relaxing. What is worse, the light emitted by their screens will trick your mind into thinking that it is daytime and therefore cause you to stay alert and awake. It is better to turn them all off at least one hour before bed.

If you have any phone calls or e-mails that you need to make before hitting the hay, you should also handle them all at least 3 hours before bed. Any later than that and you will reduce your chances of falling asleep naturally. After all, you should not underestimate the power of getting lost in a conversation. If you constantly communicate with someone before bedtime, inform them that you"digitally detach"yourself within a specific hour; chances are, they will respect your decision.

Relax your body and mind.

Now that you are cleansed, nourished and have everything put together for tomorrow, you can indulge in some relaxing activities to really lull you to sleep. There are countless ways to relax yourself, but if you are stumped for ideas, here are some great suggestions:

Read a light novel. This is a tricky suggestion, because it may cause you to lose even more hours of sleep if the novel is so engaging. However, most people tend to fall asleep while reading a fun yet not really thought-provoking story. You can also consider reading a textbook. It would be a miracle if it will not knock you out after a few pages.

Listen to an audiobook. Remember the time when your mom or dad read to you in bed when you were little? You can recreate this in a way by listening to an audiobook. This would probably be even better than reading a novel because you can close your eyes and keep the lights off while listening.

Meditate or do progressive muscle relaxation. These will help put your body into a state of deep relaxation. This is the best time to try the ones described in the previous Chapter.

Meditate or write in a journal. The best way to reduce stress from your mind is by praying, meditating, or unleashing it all on the pages of your journal. These strategies are incredibly powerful when it comes to letting go of anxiety. Try keeping a journal next to your bed and then jot down whatever crosses your mind for a few minutes. You can also make voice memos if you are not in the mood to write but would still like to express your thoughts into words. Don't forget to delete them afterwards, if you feel that there is a need to do so.

Slip on some fuzzy socks and a seamed cap. This may sound silly, but it is actually incredibly relaxing to wear socks and a seamed cap (otherwise called a beanie) in bed. Even the National Sleep Foundation supports this, because according to the researchers, the socks cause the blood vessels to expand. This will then signal the brain that the body is ready to sleep.

Now switch off the lights, get nice and warm underneath your blanket, and enjoy the cool and relaxing ambiance of your bedroom. Enjoy the state of "quiet wakefulness" and entertain yourself with an imaginative story, which will weave into a real dream. Before you know it, you are fast asleep.

Chapter 23: Getting In The Sleep Mindset

Having considered sleep disorders in the last chapter, there is now the opportunity to consider what else may be affecting your ability to sleep well. It may well be that, even if you do have an underlying medical condition, or show some of the signs of some of the disorders mentioned above, you will still be able to make some progress by ensuring that you are as best prepared as you can be for trying to get to sleep – and staying asleep for the optimum amount of time.

In some ways, the journey you have gone on already in picking up and reading this book means that you want to make some changes. We have talked already of knowing your own mind and body, but it is not remiss to emphasise again how important it is to understand what situations you are in when you do feel fully rested – it might seem like a fuss, but your physiological make-up requires that you sleep every day, so you have plenty of experiment material! Once you are better aware of your own requirements, the next step is to try to get into a mind-set that you are going to do something about it – and this also includes ensuring you are in the best place mentally that you can be to allow sleep to come more naturally and easily We will consider practical solutions later, but for now, are you able to take a few moments to think of two or three things that you could do to try and get some more sleep, or a more restful night of sleep.

The chances are you said "well I just have to get to bed earlier" – that may well be the case, but the chances are too that you tell yourself that most nights anyway, then find yourself still awake when you know you should be asleep! Don't be too hard on yourself – we all do it – we think we deserve just that bit more time to ourselves, or another episode of that superb television box set – we have earned it after a hard day haven't we? Of course this is fine from time to time, but if it starts getting into a bad habit then you may have a problem on your hands.

Perhaps you have told yourself that you really must try and not look at electronic devices before you go to sleep – you may have heard stories about the certain type of light emanating from these, and the fact that this is thought to impact on some people as to how quickly they can fall asleep, and the type of sleep that they then have. There certainly seems to be some truth in this concept – not least based on the principle that looking at such bright devices late at night, and particularly in the dark, can influence your body clock – perhaps delaying the onset of sleep. There is, of course, a danger of how such activities may affect your eyesight, but that is another conversation. Devices such as smartphones and tablets can then, experts believe affect your sleep. "It is very hard" I hear you say.

Indeed that is true – these types of devices are absolutely everywhere these days – it is just so easy to quickly check what is going on with your social media feeds – you wouldn't want to be the last to know something, or for a conversation with a friend to be missed. For the younger generation, this is how things have always been – they have grown up not knowing a world where such devices were not part of the normal – however that does not mean they are not having an impact. For the older generations, these sorts of devices are new – maybe they were more used to reading a book or magazine in bed before going to sleep, and perhaps later they started to watch TV before trying to sleep – either in another room, or in their bedroom. Screens of any kind are likely to have an effect, however it is the particular type of light from smartphones and tablet devices which are thought to have most impact.

Conclusion

Getting a good night's rest is one of the basic needs of your existence and this condition can impact your sleep pattern. This disorder can create havoc in your life as it may make you feel sleepy throughout the day and leave you feeling restless. It can also trigger migraines in some people, which do not let them function normally.

I hope that after reading this book, you are now better equipped to understand this condition and possibly tackle it. I have listed many different types of treatments for this condition. Hopefully you choose one that suits your condition and your lifestyle the best.

Each one of us has the ability to overcome even the deadliest of diseases with sheer determination, and Sleep Apnea is no exception to this rule. I request all of you who are suffering from sleep disorders to take a step and help yourself by opting for one of the treatments listed in this book. You can discuss these with your physician or specialist and find out what will work best for you.

CPSIA information can be obtained
at www.ICGtesting.com
Printed in the USA
BVHW041807240221
600781BV00011B/364

9 781990 268373